Aesthetic Dentistry
With Indirect Resins

Howard Stean

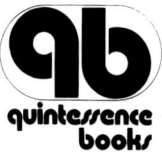

Quintessence Publishing Co., Inc. 1992
Chicago, London, Berlin, São Paulo and Tokyo

First published 1992 by
Quintessence Publishing Company Ltd
London, UK

© 1992 Quintessence Publishing Co. Ltd

British Library Cataloguing in Publication Data

Stean, Howard
  Aesthetic Dentistry with Indirect Resins
  I. Title
  617.6

ISBN 1-85097-026-2

Printed and bound in Great Britain by
Butler & Tanner Ltd, Frome, Somerset
from typesetting by Alacrity Phototypesetters,
Banwell Castle, Weston-super-Mare

Contents

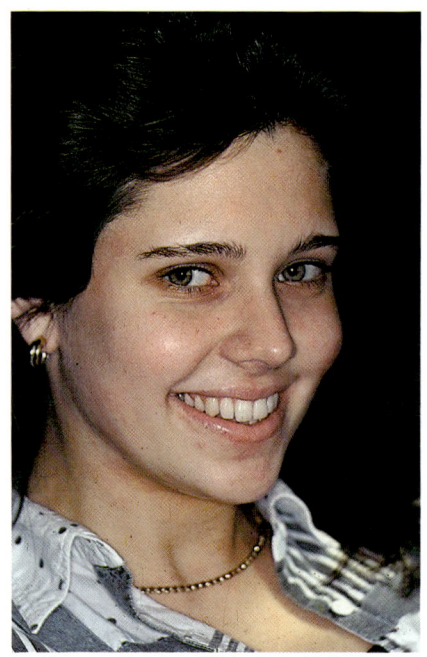

A natural "aesthetic" smile is available to those who seek it.

Foreword

Aesthetic dentistry, long-shunned by more conservative practitioners as being unimportant and only 'cosmetic' in nature, has matured into a legitimate and highly important part of dentistry. When considering the overall psychological health and well-being of dental patients, some practitioners and many patients have concluded that aesthetic dentistry may be more significant than those traditional aspects primarily concerned with the treatment of pain, disease and dysfunction.

Numerous challenges face practitioners of aesthetic dentistry. One of the most important is keeping up-to-date with the innumerable new products and techniques that are routinely introduced onto the market. Some have long since given up their attempts to keep abreast of new developments and have merely carried on using concepts of the past, while others have accumulated new information, developed new procedures, and applied them to dental practice and the service of patients.

Howard Stean is a highly motivated and innovative practitioner, researcher and student of dentistry. He has put together a combination of pragmatic and clinical information, integrated with the most up-to-date research references from around the world. This book is descriptive, well-illustrated with examples from his own cases, thought-provoking and most importantly, useful to those interested in practising the concepts of current aesthetic restorative dentistry.

GORDON J. CHRISTENSEN, DDS, MSD, PhD
Founder and Senior Consultant,
Clinical Research Associates.

5

Acknowledgements

I owe a considerable debt of gratitude to my technicians, *Complete Crown and Bridge* for their unstinting help and support, in particular Bill Milton and Nick Powers.

Also, I would like to thank Gary Unterbrink, Technical Director of Ivoclar-Vivadent Lichtenstein for his invaluable clinical advice, and Ron Freeman and Allan Budgen of Ivoclar-Vivadent UK for their encouragement and advice.

Finally, my thanks must go to Ellen Williams for help with typing the manuscript, editorial assistance and patience through the project.

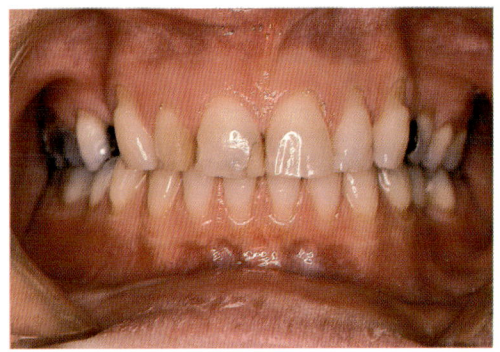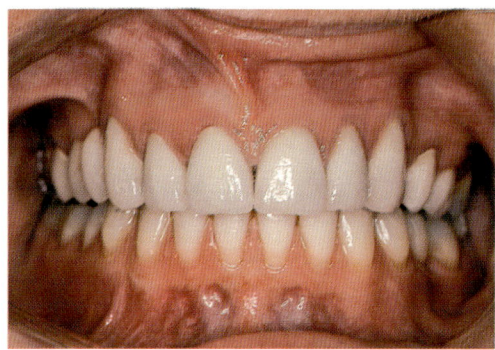

A major reconstruction was necessary to meet this patient's aesthetic requirements.

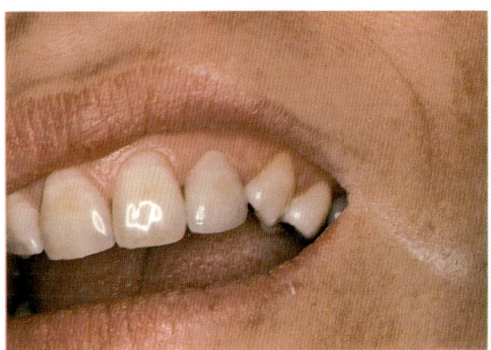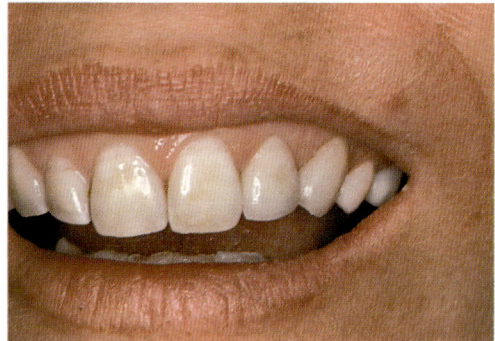

This patient was concerned with a single dental irregularity.

From the smallest blemish to the most extensive reconstruction, the importance of each particular problem to the patient must be given full consideration.

Introduction

In dentistry, as in other disciplines, a pent up demand for "cosmetic" improvements is being unleashed. The advent of genuinely new technical advances now enable most, if not all, dental defects to be rectified, whilst at the same time preserving the original dentition. A natural "aesthetic" smile is available to those who seek it.

The scope for improvement is so great that it is limited purely by the ingenuity and enthusiasm of the clinician. But it is not for the dentist to decide what is important to improve, for the patient is the arbiter of good taste in this very personal matter. Nevertheless, no distinction can be made between so-called cosmetic dentistry and good conservative dentistry. All proper dental treatment should be aesthetic. Any dentist who chooses to ignore this inevitable trend does so at the risk of success to his practice.

This book demonstrates how the advent of the indirect resin system has extended the range of restorative possibilities and can now take its place alongside existing materials in enabling durable and aesthetic restorations to be routinely carried out.

Many treatment plans call for the replacement of missing teeth and also the restoration of the remaining dentition. Indirect resin is a useful additional material that may be considered in many of these cases. A single shade guide can ensure that all the restorations are properly matched and this fact alone is of great assistance in helping to re-create an aesthetic result.

Isosit/Concept Indirect Resin Material
The restorations described in this book are based on the use by the author of the indirect resin material, Isosit/Concept, which is produced by Ivoclar-Vivadent. The author has used this material for a considerable number of cases over the past five years and has selected for this book cases which he feels are of particular significance.

Two Types of Material Available
For intra coronal use the indirect resin material SR-Isosit inlay/onlay (Concept in the USA) is available. This micro filled material is quite heavily filled and is available in seven shades. The practical use of this material in restorations is dealt with in the first section of the book (Chapters 1 to 5).

For extra coronal use — crown and bridge work, laminate veneers etc — a less heavily filled material, Chromasit, is available. This material was previously called SR Isosit N and is particularly suitable for crown and bridge work, temporary crowns and veneers. Its use is described in the second part of the book (Chapters 6 to 10).

This material can also be utilized in removable prostheses as custom made

9

denture teeth in tight space situations and in conjunction with stock denture teeth of the same shade and material.

Colour Matching

Both indirect resin materials and the porcelain materials produced by Ivoclar-Vivadent are matched to the Chromascop shade guide, thus making it possible to use all three materials in the same mouth. In this way, simple or complex treatment plans are able to be compiled in the knowledge that the precise matching of shades and materials is assured.

Experience in Use

The indirect resin system was introduced in 1976 and has been widely used during the intervening period. During this time a substantial body of clinical experience has been built up on the endurance of inlays, onlays and crowns. Research is ongoing, and all the results tend to show that indirect cured resin is a durable and versatile material.

The reader is encouraged to refer to the standard works on restorative dentistry (a short list of recommended books is given below) and use this book as an adjunct to the well-tried and accepted techniques.[1][2][3][4][5]

All of the cases referred to and illustrated in this volume were treated by the author in a London based general practice.

As with most general practices, a wide range of treatment methods is used but the indirect resin system has been particularly successful for selected cases since first introduced some four years ago.

References

1 Levin, E. (1978) Dental esthetics and the golden proportions. J. Prosthet. Dent. 40:244.
2 Lombardi, R. (1973) The principles of visual perception and their clinical application to denture esthetics. J. Prosthet. Dent. 29:358.
3 Lombardi, R. (1977) Factors mediating against excellence in dental esthetics. J. Prosthet. Dent. 38:243.
4 Lacy, A.M. (1987) JADA vol. 114, p.257-.
5 Christensen, G.J. (1989) Int. Dent. J. 39, 155-161.

Suggested further reading

Rufenacht, Claude R. (1990) Fundamentals of esthetics. Quintessence.
Goldstein, R. (1976) Esthetics in dentistry. Lippincott.
Jordan, R. (1988) Esthetic composite bonding. Decker.
Scharer, Rinn and Koff. (1982) Esthetic Guidelines for restorative dentistry. Quintessence.
Shillingburg, Jacobi and Brackett. (1987) Fundamentals of tooth preparations. Quintessence.
Smith, B. (1990) Planning and making crowns and bridges. Martin Dunitz.

Chapter 1

Indirect Resins: A New Concept

Material for the indirect resin system has been developed from a need to enhance the clinical performance of light-cured resins in order to create a restorative material that would offer a longer term durability together with good aesthetics.[1] [2]

Whilst light-curing (direct) composite resins have established their place in restorative dentistry and offer an instant and aesthetic solution to many cases, their short-comings have become only too obvious. In Table 1-1 a list of well-known problems that are still encountered with light-cured resins is shown and compared with a newer material, in the indirect resin system.

Indirect resins utilise a two-stage technique. This permits the dental technician to produce an inlay (or onlay) that is stronger, more dimensionally stable, and more durable than any self-cured composite. Only in the laboratory can polymerisation at 120°C and 6 bar pressure be attained. The result is a non-porous, homogenous restoration that is ready for insertion. Indirect resins are not intended as a replacement for all light-cured restorations but they do offer excellent aesthetics combined with a superior strength that gives more durable restorations.[13] [14]

The resin material is a dedicated urethane dimethacrylate with a highly loaded filler of 56% volume (74% by weight). It is a homogeneous microfilled material.

It is accepted that direct resins continue to have many indications in restorative dentistry and, generally speaking, are more suited to smaller cavities and situations where loading is not high.[15] Examples will be shown where direct resin fillings would be difficult to accomplish and where the indirect system offers real advantages.

Whilst indirect resins can be cured by various methods: by chemical catalyst, by light, heat or by a combination of heat and pressure, this book describes the applications of indirect resin formed by heat and pressure (Ivoclar/Vivadent). This product is available in two versions which are designed to deal with the various clinical demands encountered in restorative dentistry.

Broadly speaking the intra-coronal uses are met by the Inlay/Onlay material (eg SR-ISOSIT). The extra-coronal material (eg Chromasit) which is less highly filled is designed for veneers and crown and bridgework with metal substructures. Table 1-2 shows the physical values of indirect (heat/pressure cured) resin compared with the physical values of a typical direct resin.

It is important to understand that the chemical composition of indirect resin material belies its clinical performance. The laboratory process that is a part of

TABLE 1-1

Comparison of Clinical Problems associated with Direct and Indirect Resin Materials

Direct (Composite) Resin	*Indirect Resin*
Polymerisation shrinkage leading to open contacts.[3][4][5][6] Danger of porosity leading to voids	Laboratory processed restoration is dimensionally stable and eliminates any porosity
Variable rates of wear in clinical use leading to restrictions on applications in posterior regions	Hard surface that exhibits a wear rate comparable to natural tooth substance
Micro-leakage around margins with attendant problems, such as staining, secondary caries and adverse pulpal responses[7]	Much reduced micro-leakage
Curing may produce undesirable stresses[8][9]	Minimal adverse effects as only a small layer of bonding resin is needed
Plucking of filler particles from the surface causes a rough surface (not applicable to microfill resins)	Homogeneous microfilled material does not permit this effect to occur
Difficulties in producing the desired contour 'freehand'	Any required design can be fabricated in the laboratory and returned ready to finish
Change in colour on polymerisation — causing difficulties in colour matching	Laboratory processed material is colour-stable — customised shade tabs enable accurate colour matching. Can be adjusted and repolished easily in the mouth and can be repaired with composite resin just as easily

TABLE 1-2

Physical Properties of Indirect Resin Compared with a Direct Resin

	Indirect Resin Material		*Direct Resin*
	SR-Isosit	*Chromasit*	*Heliomolar*
tensile strength	90-120 N/mm²	80 N/mm²	70-80 N/mm²
deformation at 200 MPa	3.5-4.5%	25%	8-9%
Vickers hardness 0.5/30	500-600 N/mm²	145 N/mm²	360-410 N/mm
E-modulus N/mm²	7000-10000	4000	4000-5500

TABLE 1-3

**Physical Properties of Extra Coronal Indirect Resin
Compared with Natural Tooth Substance**

	Enamel	Ceramic	Chromasit
Vickers Hardness N/mm^2	ca. 2 800	ca. 6 000	ca. 200
Modulus of Elasticity N/mm^2	ca. 47 000	ca. 60 000	ca. 4 000
Compressive strength	ca. 410	ca. 180	ca. 500

the system converts the resin into an altogether different substance, in the sense that its physical properties are improved greatly. The density and homogenity are increased and all voids are eliminated. The high pressure and temperature improves the strength and removes porosity. Table 1-3 shows the physical properties compared with enamel and ceramic.

Compared with acrylic used in crown and bridgework, indirect resin is much stronger with better wear resistance. Another important feature of indirect resin is that it is a microfilled material and like other microfilled composites it can achieve a very high degree of polish which can be maintained in clinical use. It can also be re-polished after alterations time and time again to the same lustre, which is an important feature. This very shiny surface is kind to tissues, and in clinical practice there seems to be acceptance of polished indirect resin by the gingival tissues with minimal inflammatory response. A study by Strohaver[16] noted that heat/pressure cured resin contains less voids than porcelain.

Clinical wear of indirect resin

A recent study by David James[17] rated heat/pressure cured resin highly in a three year clinical survey and a more recent study by Mitchem[18] compared wear rates with direct resins over a five year period. The indirect resin (Isosit/ Concept) had the lowest wear rate, which was less than the direct filling material that exhibited the lowest wear rate of all the direct materials tested. (Fig 1-1.)

It is also interesting to note that the wear rate diminished during the study period, which may lead to the speculation that longer term wear could be even lower. The extra-coronal system has also been fully evaluated, and a study by the University of Alabama demonstrated that resin bonded crowns wore at approximately 7 microns per year. This figure is of the same order as the wear rate of natural tooth substance.

A further clinical study[19] over a four year period rated 91 out of 92 inlays as clinically satisfactory. The only unsatisfactory inlay was the first made and this may have been due to a lack of clinical experience in handling the material.

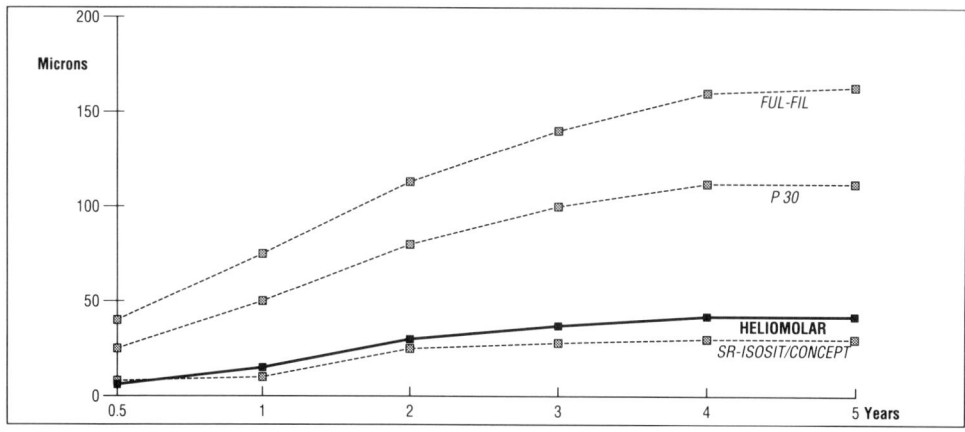

Fig 1-1 Clinical Wear. Comparison of an indirect resin with three direct resins.

Resin cement: an integral part of the system

The dual-curing resin cement is an integral feature of the entire concept of indirect inlays and onlays. Unlike traditional inlays of gold the indirect system does not require a close fit of the inlay to the cavity. In fact, a tight fit is undesirable, because sufficient space is necessary for adequate bonding. The strong bond achieved between tooth, cement, and restoration contributes to the increased strength of the restored tooth.

The resin cement is a lightly filled microfill composite resin formulated to bond to the tooth and adhere firmly to the fitting surface of resin inlays and onlays, veneers and crowns. It is supplied in a two paste system that is both chemically and light cured (Dual cure cement). Polymerisation will therefore begin upon mixing and will eventually become complete. The use of light curing with an effective light source will hasten curing and the time curve makes this procedure mandatory in clinical practice.

As with direct composite restorations a certain degree of wear is likely and it would be expected that a microfill structure would exhibit less wear than a macrofill material. Resin cements are, in fact, available in differing formulations, depending upon the manufacturer. Recent work by Ariyaratnam, et al[20] shows cement thicknesses of 15 to 90 microns in fitted inlays.

The acid-etched enamel tooth margins (Fig 1-2) and cavity lining is utilised as a bonding surface for the cement. The heat and pressure cured resin of the inlays is fully polymerised and no free radicals are available for true chemical

14

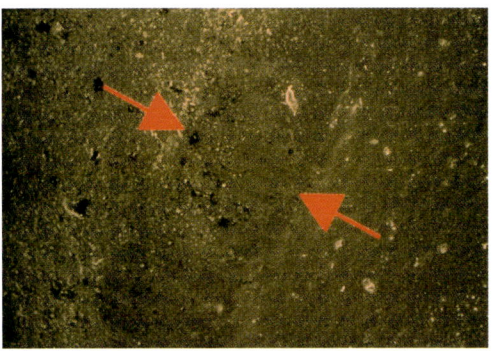

Fig 1-2 A highly magnified view of the cement margin (indicated by arrows) after 2.5 years.

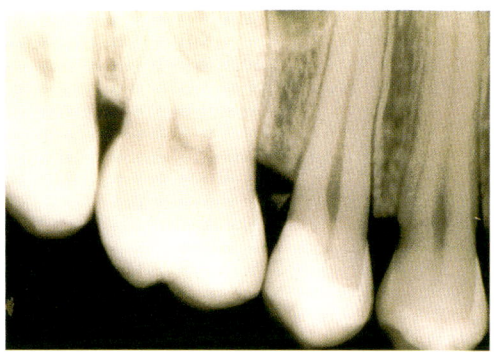

Fig 1-3 Inlay is radio-opaque, permitting inspection of marginal fit. Notice also the distal fragment of cement.

bonding. Nevertheless, resin cement attaches securely to resin inlays and onlays, and cement failure does not occur. A special bonding liquid (Special Bond II) is available to increase bonding strength of the cement to the resin but this is generally only indicated when fixing laminate veneers. The advent of satisfactory dentine adhesives has enabled resin restorations to be attached directly to non-enamel surfaces as well. This feature is useful when additional retention is required, such as in the fixation of laminate veneers where a full enamel face is absent. The use of dentine adhesives is described in Chapter 7.

The cement phase of traditional inlays and crowns is well known as being the weakest link in the finished restorations, and so it is correct to address this question to the resin cement in the indirect resin system. Careful monitoring of completed restorations over several years is the only sure way of determining the long term success. The introduction

of ultrasound techniques may point the way towards the use of higher-filled resins for cementation of inlays.[21]

More studies are needed to evaluate the long term endurance of restorations made in indirect resin and the marginal integrity is one obvious area that should be examined.

Comparison with other restorative materials

Silver amalgam
This has been, and still continues to be widely used as a restorative material. There can be no doubt of its potential as an effective medium-to-long-term material when properly handled. It is only recently that questions have been raised regarding the possible harmful effects to the patient due to its mercury content. The latest research has not shown conclusive findings on this aspect of amalgam. The introduction of a newer gallium-based amalgam will side-step this problem area.

TABLE 1-4

Comparison of Porcelain and Indirect Resin for Inlays

Porcelain	Indirect Resin
Bulk of the final restoration needs to be carefully appraised: a minimum thickness of 1 mm and a maximum thickness of 2.5 mm should be produced, otherwise fracture can occur	Suitable for a wide range of cavity designs, minimum thickness of 1 mm to 1.5 mm for cuspal coverage: there is no maximum thickness
Careful checks needed to ensure that no lateral excursive movements are on porcelain due to·the potential for aggressive tooth wear of the opposing tooth	Wear rate of the opposing tooth is negligible
Inlay material does not wear	Wear rate of approx. 7 microns per year corresponds to natural tooth substance
Difficult to repolish in the mouth	Easy to repolish to a high lustre
Excellent tissue acceptance	Excellent tissue acceptance

From an aesthetic standpoint, amalgam is probably the most unattractive material to choose. Apart from the metallic appearance, which gradually blackens in the mouth, the internal tooth staining that amalgam creates can pose serious problems for the restorative dentist (see Chapter 3). One purpose of this book is to illustrate how teeth can be durably and aesthetically restored. Therefore a case can be made for restricting the use of amalgam to situations where good appearance is less important than structural repair.

Porcelain inlays

Another offshoot from the technological advances that created porcelain veneers is that of etched porcelain inlays. As with indirect resin inlays, porcelain inlays offer good, aesthetically pleasing fillings that, in the correct circumstances, are durable. Important differences between indirect resin material and porcelain are summarised in Table 1-4. However, newer cast and milled porcelains are now being introduced which will, to a large extent, overcome the limitations posed by traditional materials.

Gold

Were it not for its appearance, gold might remain the closest to the ideal restorative material. It is strong, adaptable, and above all has stood the test of time as a most durable dental restorative. Where appearance is not important, gold continues to be the material of choice for long term restorations. Gold may also be selected when a potentially unstable occlusion would result from use of a softer material such as amalgam or indirect resin.

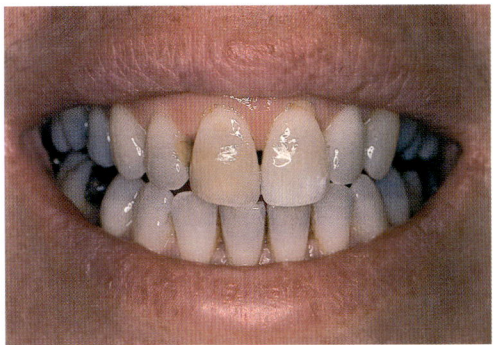

Fig 1-4 Patient demanded an aesthetic improvement.

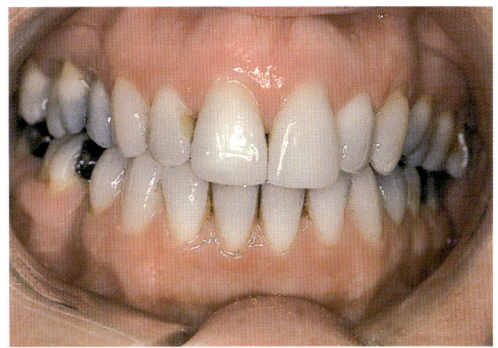

Fig 1-5 Two laminate Veneers were fitted. Note the excellent tissue condition.

Periodontal considerations

A basic tenet of all dentistry is to avoid damage to the tissues. Unfortunately it is all too easy to produce adverse changes in the supporting tissues by inserting poorly shaped and finished restorations. Any incursion into the gingival crevice carries with it the risk of periodontal damage. Indirect resin restorations offer two distinct advantages that could lessen the risk of periodontal damage. Firstly, the laboratory processed and finished inlays and onlays are returned ready for fitting. They are contoured properly by the technician, removing one clinical procedure that could be imperfectly executed. Upon cementa tion final polishing of the margin can easily be carried out with graded silicone polishing cups.

Secondly, the margins need not be extended sub-gingivally unless tooth structure is deficient in that area. Indirect resin material is etch-bonded to tooth with a dual-cured resin cement: tooth material need not be cut away to secure retention. Newer dentine adhesion systems can also be used to enhance retention when enamel is deficient.

Extra-coronal restorations such as labial (laminate) veneers also seem to be associated with excellent gingival health (Fig 1-4 and 1-5). This great advance in aesthetic, minimum intervention dentistry is covered in Chapter 7.

Caution

No restorative material can confer protection against periodontal damage when incorrectly used. It is incumbent on every dentist to take every precaution to prepare a healthy supporting environment before starting restorative treatment. The ease with which indirect resin restorations can be placed should not lure the operator into a false sense of security.

Occlusal considerations

Without a working knowledge of the principles of occlusion any attempt at restorative dentistry will result in the occasional unpleasant surprise and failure. The same principles need to be applied when indirect resin restorations are planned. It is generally accepted that there are two approaches to choose from: the *conformist* and the *reorganised*.

In the *conformist* method a single, or perhaps more than one tooth is restored without any attempt to alter the pre-existing occlusal relationship in the mouth. The assumption is made that the patient is comfortable in his, or her, pattern of occlusal behaviour. The restoration should "fit in" and conform to the occlusal pattern. This does not mean neglecting to reduce over-erupted cusps that may impinge on the new restoration and risk fracture or other complications. It does mean that the new restoration will not cause any disturbance of the occlusion.

The *reorganised* approach is quite different. Here a decision is made following an analysis of the occlusion that in order to successfully treat the patient an initial occlusal alteration and improvement needs to be undertaken. A period of "settling" is then normally allowed for the "new" occlusion to become reproducable. It is suggested that initial experience with indirect resin inlays and onlays be confined to single units in the *conformist* mode.

An example of how the *conformist* approach to occlusion can simplify treatment and avoid the need to use complicated articulators is shown in Figs 1-6 to 1-8. In this case a missing upper molar is to be replaced. A pre-operative assessment of the occlusion revealed that preparation of the abutment teeth for full crowns and a three unit fixed bridge would eliminate all existing occlusal contacts in the quadrant. This would necessitate careful mounting on an adjustable articulator and some experience in dealing with occlusion. The option of making an adhesive (Maryland) bridge with an indirect resin pontic would side-step this potential problem, and permit the missing tooth to be replaced without disturbing the existing occlusal function. This is a simpler procedure. The use of indirect resin in adhesive bridgework is covered in more detail in Chapter 9.

From the above observations it should be apparent that no restorative treatment should be made before some initial assessment of the patient's occlusion has been done.

The occlusal assessment can include marking the occlusal contacts with articulating paper, and designing the inlay to avoid occlusal contacts at the margins, wherever possible. Indirect resin is easy to adjust, and wears at a rate comparable to natural tooth substance. This feature of the material can be useful. Full coverage restorations can also be made utilising indirect resin. Should a lower wear rate be desirable porcelain or metal should be selected.

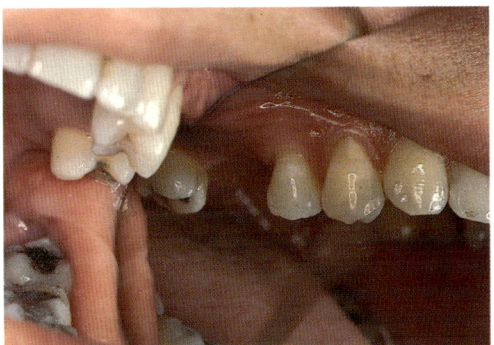

Fig 1-6 Missing molar to be replaced.

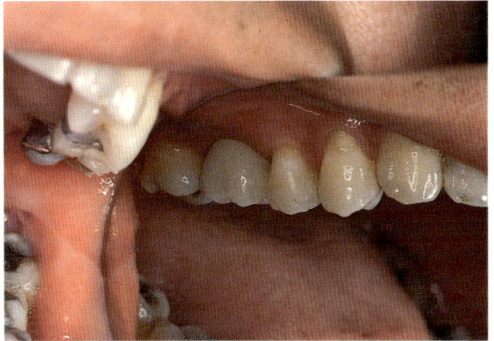

Fig 1-7 Option of Maryland bridge with indirect resin pontic was selected, rather than a fixed three unit bridge.

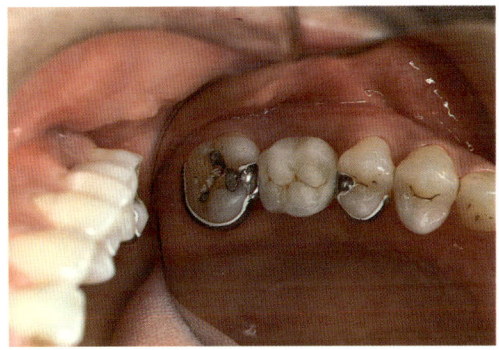

Fig 1-8 Occlusal view of finished bridge.

References

1   James, D. (1983) An esthetic inlay technique for posterior teeth. Quintessence Int. vol. 14, pp.1-7.

2   Douglas, W.H., Fields, R.P. and Fundingsland, J. (1989) Minneapolis MN J. Dent. 17:104-8.

3   Hansen, E.K. (1982) Scand. J. Dent. Res. 190:480-483.

4   McCollock, A.J. and Smith, B.G.N. (1986) Brit. Dent. J. 161:405.

5   Causton, B.E., Miller, B. and Sefton, J. (1985) Brit. Dent. J. 159:397.

6   Jones, Grieve and Youngson. (1988) J. Dent. 16:130-134.

7   Goring, R.E. (1972) Microleakage around dental restorations. JADA 84:1349.

8   Eick, J.D. and Welch, F.H. (1986) Quint. Int. 17:103-111.

9   Jensen, M.E. and Chan, D.C.N. (1985) Posterior composite resin dental restoration materials. Pub. Peter Szulc Co, p.243-262.

10   Douglas, Fields and Fundingsland. (1989) J. Dent. 17:184-188.

11   Robinson, P.B., Moore, B.K. and Swartz, M.L. (1987) Op. Dent. 12:113-116.

12   Sheth, Jensen and Sheth. (1989) Quint. Int. 20:831-836.
Garber, Goldstein and Feinman. (1988) Porcelain laminate veneers. Pub. Quintessence Books.
Caldwell, C.B. (1961) Bleaching vital or non-vital teeth. J. Calif. Dent. Ass. 42:234.
Eames, W.B. and Lodato, F.M. (1971) Evaluation of stain remover. J. Georgia Dent. Ass. 45:10.

13   Wendt, S. (1987) Quint. Int. vol. 18, no. 4.

14 Werrin, S.R., Jubach, T.S. and Johnson, B.W. (1980) Inlays and onlays: making the right decision. Quint. Int. 11 : 13.

15 Wilson, Nairn. (1991) Current status and rationale for composite inlays and onlays. Brit. Dent. J. April, 269-72.

16 Strouhauer, R.A. and Mattie, D.R. (1987) J. of Prosthet. Dent. vol. 57, no. 5, 559-565.

17 James, D. (1986) Quint. Int. Oct., no. 6916, pp.1-7.

18 Mitcham et al. (1990) J.D.R. 142, vol. 69.

19 Bishop, B.M. (1989) A heat/pressure cured composite inlay system. Aust. Prosth. J.

20 Ariyaratnam, M., Wilson, M.A., Wilson, N.H.F. and Watts, D.C. (1990) J. Rest. Dent. Nov., pp.16-18.

21 ESPE Sono cem. system: introduced 1992.

Chapter 2

Indirect Inlays

Inlay design and preparation

The concept of indirect inlays and on-lays is illustrated in the following diagrams, and also by a clinical example.

Fig 2-1 shows a common example of cusp fracture adjacent to an existing restoration. This is also shown in a typical case (Figs 2-5 to 2-8) in a tooth with a lingual carious fracture. The indirect resin inlay system offers the most conservative way of restoring this tooth.

Fig 1-2 shows how a new pinned amalgam filling would need further tooth cutting, and Fig 2-3 shows the outline of a gold inlay. An indirect resin inlay is no bigger than the original filling plus the fracture. One feature of the inlay/onlay

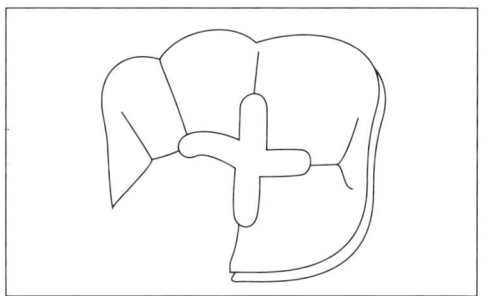

Fig 2-1 A broken cusp adjacent to an existing restoration.

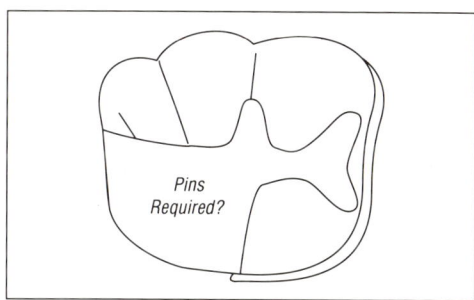

Fig 2-2 An amalgam restoration would need further tooth cutting and would probably require pinning.

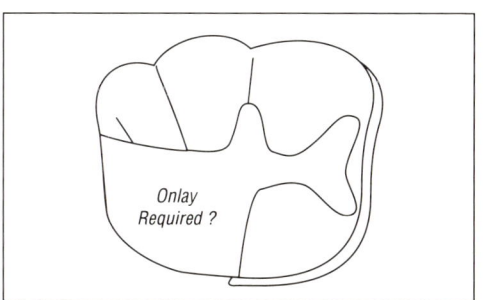

Fig 2-3 Outline of a gold inlay restoration.

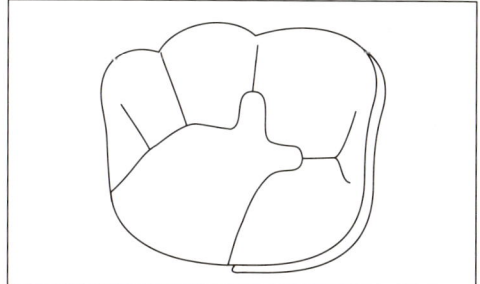

Fig 2-4 Outline of an indirect resin restoration. The restoration is no larger than the original filling plus the fracture.

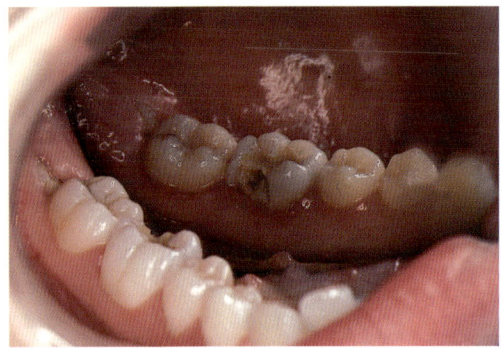

Fig 2-5 Carious tooth requires restoration.

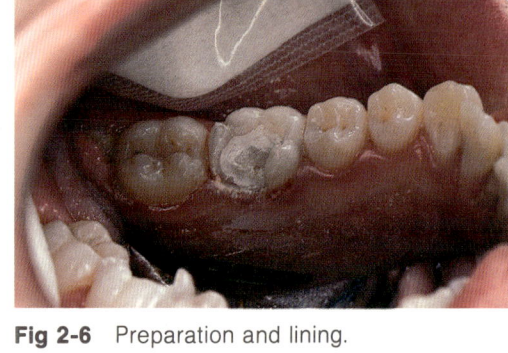

Fig 2-6 Preparation and lining.

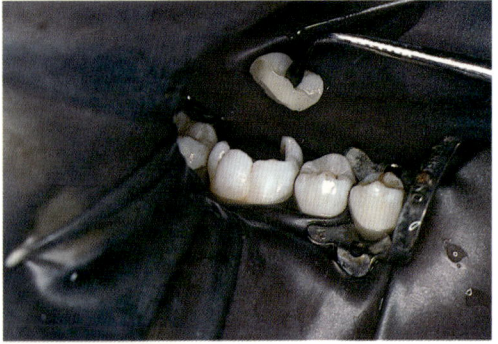

Fig 2-7 Inlay ready to try-in.

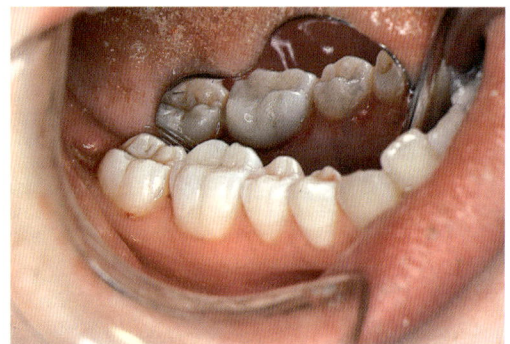

Fig 2-8 The completed case.

preparation is the preservation of what tooth substance remains. The final preparation need not extend further than the initial filling (having removed all undercuts and caries).

As the restoration is retained by a resin-bonded acid etched cement there is no need to extend the margins past the original defect. A sharp non-bevelled external margin on enamel is easily cut, whilst sharp internal angles are to be avoided, as these may induce stresses. The enamel inlay interface should ideally be 120°/60° angle. However the position of the margin relative to the cusp slope will frequently dictate the actual angle. It is important to create a butt fit with no fragile inlay margins, and no fragile enamel margins.

Cavity lining techniques for indirect resin restorations

An essential element in tooth preparation for indirect resin inlays is correct cavity lining. As with cavity design, the techniques formerly used for gold inlays and amalgam restorations are not suited for indirect resins. A rethink of the objectives and hence the lining materials is required.

The objectives for linings are:

1. Removal of all tooth undercuts that

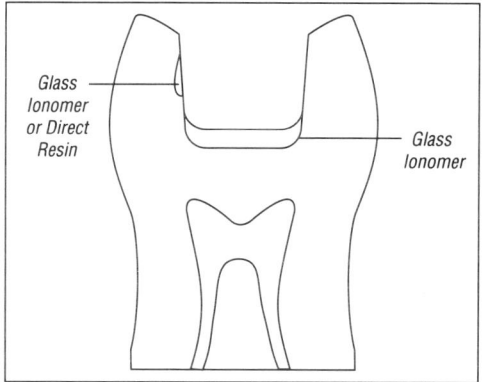

Fig 2-9 Minimal occlusal lining.

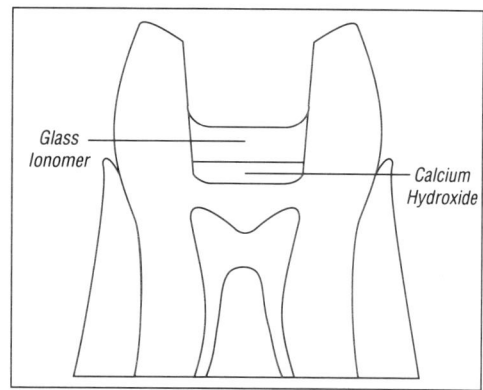

Fig 2-10 Deep occlusal lining.

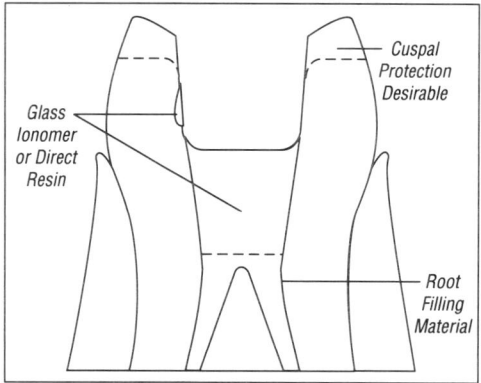

Fig 2-11 Lining for a non-vital tooth.

remain after cavity preparation. Teeth should have been prepared so that all cavity margins are on sound tooth substance. It is not necessary, or desirable, to over-prepare teeth in order to cut away all undercut areas, provided that the undercuts are capable of being removed by lining.

2. The lining should provide adequate pulpal protection when vital teeth are being restored.

3. The lining, or 'core' in non-vital teeth should be adequately retained.

4. Lining material adjacent to outer tooth walls should not block light transmission. The phenomenon of 'colour coupling' relies on light transmission between the cemented inlay and the tooth. This subject is covered in greater detail in Chapter 3.

5. Linings should be chemically compatible with the resin material and the cement system. A strong bond between the lining and cement will improve the retention of the inlay, provided that the lining material also has

a strong bond to the dentine of the tooth.

From a perusal of these requirements it will be apparent that traditional linings such as zinc phosphate and zinc oxide/eugenol are unsuited to the indirect resin technique and should not be used.

The following three examples illustrate the correct lining techniques for different types of teeth.

Fig 2-9 shows the minimum requirement for lining a shallow occlusal cavity on a vital tooth. The occlusal floor is lined with a glass ionomer cement. Undercuts may be lined out with either direct (composite) resin or glass ionomer.

Fig 2-10 shows the lining requirement for a deeper cavity on a vital tooth. An underlining of calcium hydroxide is covered with glass ionomer.

In Fig 2-11 a non-vital tooth lining requires structural consideration. Glass ionomer or direct resin can be used and this is covered in greater detail in Chapter 8.

The advent of light cured glass ionomer and calcium hydroxide liners has made lining quick and simple. Both glass ionomer and resin will form bonds to resin cement. The surface layer of light cured calcium hydroxide liners (such as 'Basic') will also adhere to resins, thus making the system compatible in all its elements.

Impression taking

The indirect resin system is so called because an impression is required for the fabrication of a model from which the inlay is formed. Any elastomeric impression material that enables the technician to pour two good models without it tearing is suitable. The opposing arch impression can be made with alginate. Taking impressions for indirect restorations is easy as preparations are frequently supra-gingival and retraction cord need be used only when the margins are sub-gingival.

Temporization for indirect resins

A simple and effective temporary restoration can be made using a light cured temporary inlay material (eg Fermit). This temporary inlay is quick and easy to fabricate and is also easy to remove at the second clinical appointment. Any material can be selected that provides adequate strength and that can be removed completely without risk of damage to the cavity margins.

The view that eugenol-containing materials inhibit successful bonding of resins has recently been challenged (Christensen 1991[1]). Whilst it still seems that eugenol liners are unacceptable and should not be used, the chemical activity is probably short-term. Any temporary material that fulfills the requirements would therefore be acceptable. The acid-etch procedure that is routinely adopted as part of the pre-cementation of indirect inlays and onlays will, it is claimed, remove any traces of eugenol.

The technical appendix at the back of the book explains the process that is followed by the laboratory. Indirect resin material can be fabricated to colour match the tooth to be restored using a shade from the basic guide containing 7 shades. This system allows teeth to be

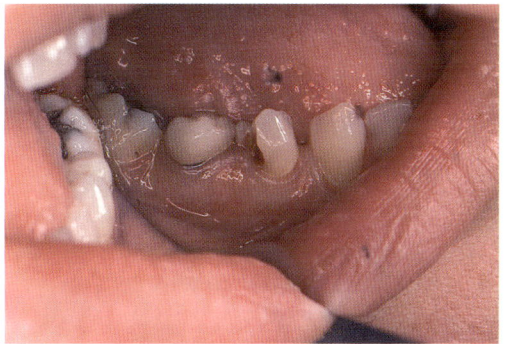

Fig 2-12 Buccal caries on a premolar.

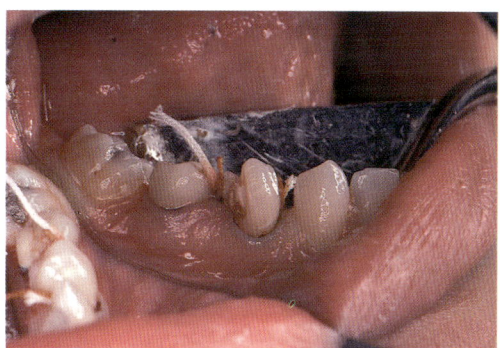

Fig 2-13 The twin cord technique in use.

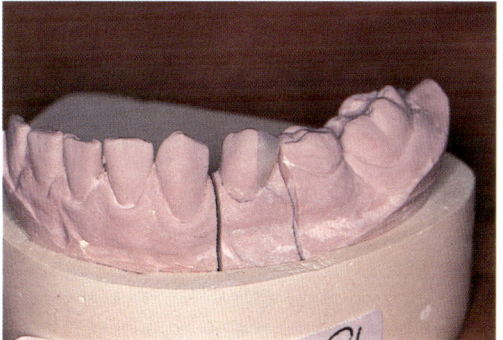

Fig 2-14 Inlay on stone model.

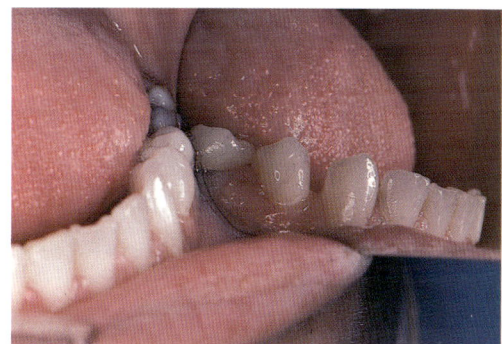

Fig 2-15 The completed restoration.

restored aesthetically, that is, to re-semble the natural tooth. Indirect resin material is an excellent substance for restoring cavities when the amount of tooth loss is extensive.

The case shown in Figs 2-12 to 2-15, and all other cases in this book, are actual patients who have been treated by the author in a general practice and show a variety of clinical indications for the use of indirect resin inlays.

Single restorations

Fig 2-12 shows extensive buccal caries on a vital premolar. The tooth loss ex-tends to the occlusal surface, and the

additional hardness of cured resin offers the possibility of a more durable restora-tion than if a light-cured resin were selected. Additionally the inlay can be well-contoured by the technician, and it is simple to execute.

At the first clinical appointment, pa-tients will appreciate a painless tech-nique which can easily be accomplished by the use of an effective topical anaes-thetic followed by adequate local an-aesthesia.

The cavity is prepared with rounded internal angles, with an inlay type pre-paration without undercuts. Bevelling is not advisable. One suitable bur is a 557 carbide bur, another smaller bur is the

169. Medium grit diamonds (bullet and flame) are also useful. As with all conservative dentistry all vital teeth should be prepared using copious water cooling. It is also advisable to keep the prepared teeth wet during all the subsequent procedures leading up to the final impression. Dehydration of dentine during operative stages is one cause of post-operative pain. A gentle but effective gingival retraction should be made wherever there are subgingival margins and an excellent method is the use of two cords (Fig 2-13). A very thin haemostatic cord is covered by a thicker non-impregnated cord. Both cords should be carefully removed before making the impression. At this stage a thorough washing out of all traces of retraction cord chemicals should be done. Styptics can cause sensitivity around necks of teeth.

Any modern elastomeric impression material can be used for the impression, and it is important to remember that the laboratory method should entail the pouring-up of two models. The impression material should therefore be capable of surviving at least two pourings without tearing. A simple inlay such as this may require only a partial impression. All other inlays should be captured with a full-mouth impression. Alginate may be used for the opposing arch impression.

On the second clinical appointment the temporary inlay is removed and the restoration is then tried in its position. It will have come from the technician in a foam-filled box, protected from damage during transit. The restoration will have been correctly contoured and finished, ready for trial insertion. The contacts should be checked using floss, and tight contacts eased carefully using a marking material. The occlusion should also be checked at this stage.

Scrupulous cleanliness needs to be observed at every stage. After adjustments the restoration needs to be degreased and cleaned and etching acid is the best method. It is more effective than alcohol or acetone. A prophyjet is also an aid to cleaning the pits and fissures of the restoration. This is the time to isolate the tooth. The use of rubber dam is recommended, but any method that enables complete moisture control is satisfactory. The cavity is then cleaned with E.D.T.A. or polyacrylic acid (Dentine Conditioner), and then washed with water. These chemicals clean and remove the smear layer on dentine. A dentine adhesive, such as 'Syntac' will seal the dentine and prevent any post insertion sensitivity.

Adequate sealing of all exposed dentine is essential to avoid post-insertion pain. A variety of factors can cause post-operative pain and sensitivity when vital teeth are being restored. Proper attention to dentine protection during this part of the indirect inlay process will prevent trouble later. Before cementation is attempted the tooth should be re-examined and any exposed vital dentine covered with a dentine sealant. This should be done even after lining. Two methods are available:

Method One Dentine Protector varnish should be applied to the clean cavity, and dried with air. This sealant should then be carefully removed from all enamel margins prior to acid etching, otherwise the etching process will be inhibited.

Method Two As an alternative to the use of Dentine Protector, the entire cavity may be coated with a thin-film dentine adhesive (eg Syntac). Intensive research and development in the field of dentine adhesion has resulted in some interesting findings. Dentine adhesive will not only improve the bond strength of resin cement to dentine but will also prevent post-operative sensitivity. The tooth margin should then be acid etched. Any convenient form of 37% phosphoric acid can be used, but it should be confined to the marginal enamel, and not spread all over the tooth. A gel type is easier to apply.

Recent research indicates that etching times as short as 15 or 30 seconds are adequate and the frosty appearance of the dried etched enamel should be self-evident. The acid must be thoroughly washed off with an air-water spray and the use of warm air to dry the tooth is to be recommended. Bond strength has been shown to be higher after drying with warm air, as opposed to cool syringe air.

The restoration is now ready for cementation. The dual cure bonding cement should be mixed in equal amounts away from bright light. An unfilled light cured resin is also applied to the tooth and cured for 10 seconds after being blown to a thin layer. Unfilled resin has been shown to provide superior wetting of the tooth surface and improved bonding via the resin tags that penetrate into the etched enamel surface.

A convenient way to insert the restoration without dropping it or contaminating it is to fix an instrument to the occlusal surface with sticky wax. The inside surface of the restoration and the cavity should both be covered with a thin film of the dual cure cement and the restoration then inserted and affixed using light pressure. The easiest way to deal with excess cement is to ensure complete removal at an early stage before curing is complete. Floss can be placed prior to placement at the gingival margin and then gently drawn through to remove the gingival excess. A short light cure of 10 seconds will partly polymerise the cement at the margins, which can then be scraped away with a sharp instrument. Whilst maintaining even, light pressure, the curing light should then be re-applied to every aspect and allowed to play on the margins for a minimum of 40 seconds per tooth surface. The dual cure cement will continue to polymerise after the light is switched off, but the restoration is ready for polishing immediately. A 12 bladed carbide finishing bur is a useful tool to adjust the occlusion, and the entire restoration can be re-finished with silicone rubber instruments.

Thirty bladed tungsten carbide burs — such as Kerr/Jet:9006 ball, 9572 straight dome, 9713 taper, 9803 bullet, and 9903/9904 needles — are also useful in finishing the margins without damaging the delicate enamel edges.

Aggressive heavy-handed finishing, and the use of blunt burs will create a 'white line'. This is evidence of damage to the margin, and could result in premature marginal failure.

Well-made indirect resins are a joy to behold (Fig 2-15): the finished teeth look perfect and patients are highly delighted with the feel and appearance.

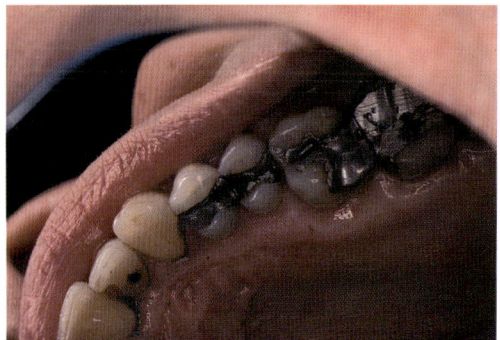

Fig 2-16   Upper quadrant to be treated.

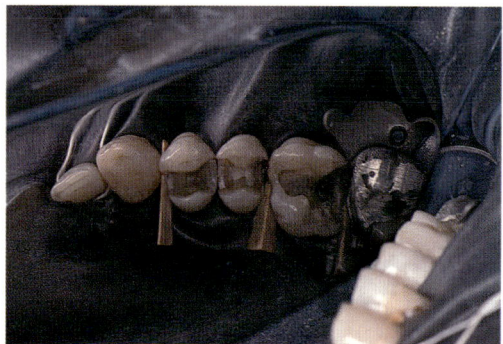

Fig 2-17   Teeth isolated and prepared.

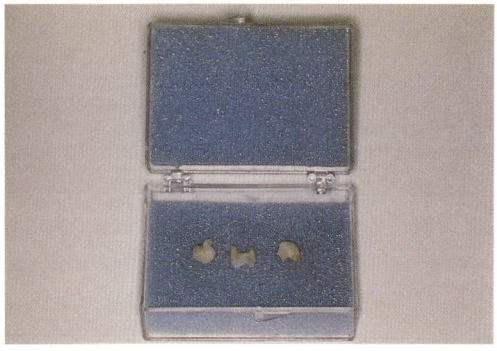

Fig 2-18   Inlays are returned in a foam lined box.

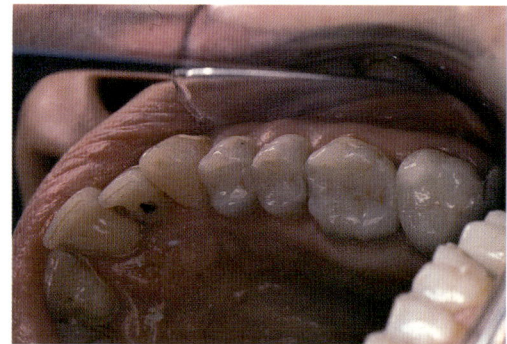

Fig 2-19   The completed case.

Multiple restorations

Multiple restorations as in Figs 2-16 to 2-19, can be prepared more readily by using a rubber dam. The employment of a rubber dam ensures excellent isolation and visibility in most restorative situations, and its use in indirect inlay procedures is helpful. Nevertheless, it is still quite possible to produce results of equal quality using alternative isolation methods when necessary.

A heavy rubber dam, well-secured with clamps and floss, offers the advantages of a completely dry field, good visibility, and also some gingival retraction. The saving in clinical time should also be considered. An entire session (preparation or cementation) can be accomplished without any break in continuity for rinsing, swallowing or conversation and this more than compensates for the time taken to apply the dam. Another simple way of achieving isolation involves the use of a pre-formed dam (Quick dam) which consists of a thinner rubber complete with a stiffened border. Upper teeth can more often be isolated easily without a dam, using either cotton rolls or a cheek pad (eg Dry tips ®).

The most sensitive part of the process in the second appointment is where the inlays are cemented in. Moisture control is essential at this stage. The acid etched margins need to be dried with warm air (a small hairdryer is recommended) and then the inlays cemented with the bonding resin, which is dual-curing. This second stage benefits immensely from the use of an effective dam.

Following isolation, the temporary fillings are removed, and vital teeth should be anaesthetised again before attempting this. The cavities should then be cleaned. Retraction cord is placed where there are gingival margins.

In this example three inlays were made to replace existing amalgam fillings (a full crown was made for the fourth tooth).

Patients are generally delighted with indirect inlays and onlays. An immediate improvement is readily appreciated, and the absence of post-operative discomfort is welcome.

Chapter 3

Aesthetic Colour Rendering

Successful aesthetic dentistry requires a different way of thinking and sustained attention to detail at every stage of the clinical process. Particular care needs to be taken to eliminate stains and marks on the tooth to be restored.

Aside from extrinsic stains caries is still the main internal cause of tooth discolouration. Whilst it is an important factor, the aesthetic restoration of teeth requires attention to all the causes of staining.

Many of these problems are associated with the consequences of existing dental work and a clear illustration of this is the staining adjacent to silver amalgam fillings. Failure to eliminate these unsightly blemishes will spoil the final result.

Staining on teeth may be external or internal. The practitioner is often presented with a combination of both types and the time to deal with these stains is at the preparation stage and not as an after-thought when inserting the final inlay.

Dealing with staining

Although a competent dental practitioner should know how to clean teeth, some helpful hints for the preparation of the enamel surface before a specialised procedure may usefully be included. A proper prophylaxis before commencing tooth preparation is essential and will also facilitate more accurate shading. Where stains remain around the margin of the prepared area they must be completely removed otherwise the final inlay will exhibit a permanent line or mark which cannot be removed.

Degradation products such as sulphides are a normal finding around amalgam fillings and this restorative material has most likely been responsible for more aesthetically compromised dentitions than many neglected mouths!

Blackish stains usually extend along the margin of the tooth — especially on the enamel — and also on the surface of the tooth, where they follow the natural crevices and pits that are sheltered from normal oral hygiene methods. (See Figs 3-1 to 3-4.)

The use of ultrasonic instruments can quickly remove these external discolourations and any remaining external staining may be removed with a jet polisher device. Another method involves the application of 37% phosphoric acid to the area, followed by careful agitation of the chemical until the stain dissolves. Surface enamel stains can also be removed using a hydrochloric-acid/pumice mixture.[1] [2]

Internal discolouration generally causes more aesthetic difficulties because the dentine, which is affected, is the prime colouring material for teeth. Internal stains are commonly present in

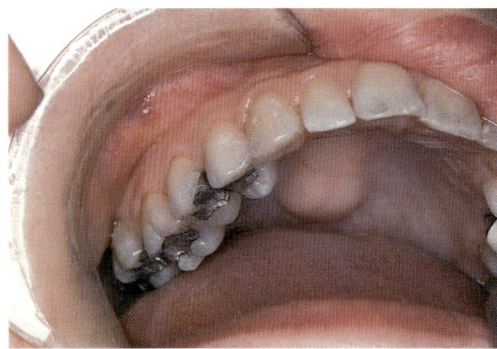

Fig 3-1 Patient requested aesthetic improvement.

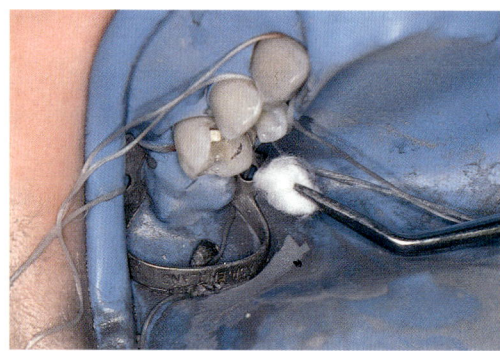

Fig 3-2 Both amalgams in the upper premolars were removed. Note the residual staining.

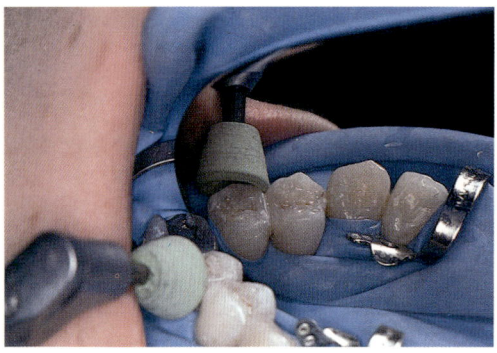

Fig 3-3 Inlays being finished with graded silicone cups.

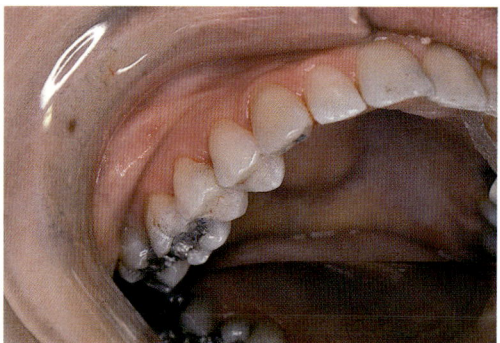

Fig 3-4 Completed case.

non-vital teeth and result from several changes including degradation of pulpal remnants, bleeding into the dentine and loss of hydration. Chemicals used in endodontic therapy can also add to the staining that is already present.

Caries is the most common cause of staining, closely followed by the treatment of it, ie silver amalgam fillings. The type and extent of stained tooth substance must be properly assessed at the treatment planning stage, if aesthetic dental restorations are to be provided. The tooth should be examined in varying types of lighting, for example with and without the operating lamp.

Light staining within the prepared cavity can be removed by applying a solution of E.D.T.A., or else polyacrylic acid (so called 'dentine conditioner') and then thoroughly washed off.

Severe and extensive internal staining is one indication for full coverage bonded crowns. Anterior teeth can now be aesthetically restored with labial (laminate) veneers and both these treatments can utilise indirect resin material.

Alternative treatment of internal staining is also possible, using vital and non-vital bleaching methods. The reader may be interested in becoming acquainted with these techniques.

Improvements in tooth colour by lightening are now becoming accepted as routine. Home bleaching should be considered as a preliminary stage in the aesthetic restoration of the mouth, before embarking upon indirect resin, or any other material.

Attention to the stain removal and cavity cleaning procedures explained above will pay off when aesthetic restorations are being made.

Note
The smear layer will inevitably be removed following thorough cleansing. This in fact, is not a significant factor when the application of a dentine adhesive is contemplated.

Although the presence of a smear layer can enhance dentine adhesion with certain products, the use of a dentine adhesive when cementing inlays and onlays is primarily concerned with the avoidance of post-operative sensitivity.

Colour matching with indirect resins

An understanding of colour is important. The practitioner needs to be thoroughly equipped with at least a basic knowledge in order to practise 'Aesthetic dentistry'. Books such as *Four Dimensional Tooth Colour System* (Muir), and *Esthetic Guidelines for Dentistry* (Scharer) are to be recommended.

It is well known that the colour of teeth comes from the dentine. The enamel does not contribute to the actual hue. This feature needs to be emulated when making aesthetic restorations, and that is why surface staining of finished restorations is not entirely satisfactory. The indirect resin material system allows for this internal colouration, and through a choice of shades is able to copy tooth colour quite well.

Colour coupling: an aesthetic concept
Intra-coronal cemented restorations permit light to pass from the adjacent tooth substance and this further improves the final appearance. By using a compatible bonding resin of the same basic material the natural tooth colour can shine through and blend with the restoration. This so called 'Colour coupling' effect offers the possibility of creating restorations that are truly concealed. This effect can be clearly demonstrated by firstly trying in an indirect inlay or onlay without any cement and noting the appearance. The restoration is then cemented with resin. A reappraisal of the result will show a marked improvement in aesthetics: the restoration will have merged with the colouration of the tooth and be less detectable.

'Colour coupling' is one reason why laminate veneers, both ceramic and resin, are able to offer better aesthetics than metal bonded ceramic (or resin) full crowns and is another reason to avoid the use of metal when attempting to restore the mouth aesthetically. A system that contains a range of translucent bonding resin shades (Heliolink) will further facilitate this blending process enabling inlays, onlays and veneers to be 'concealed' in a natural-looking smile.

Colour communication
With regard to the subject of colour communication, this area is fraught with

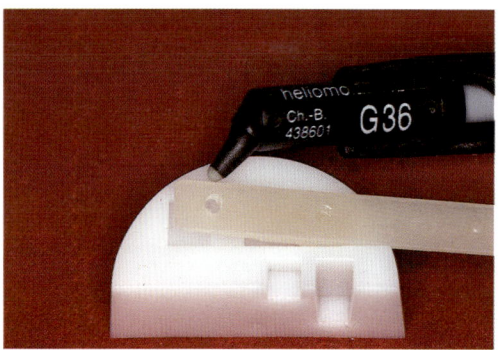

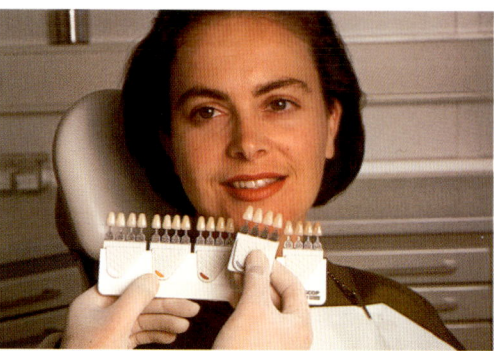

Fig 3-5 Custom made direct resin shade tabs can easily be made using a jig that is available for the purpose.

Fig 3-6 Extra-coronal restorations can be well matched using a modern shading guide system.

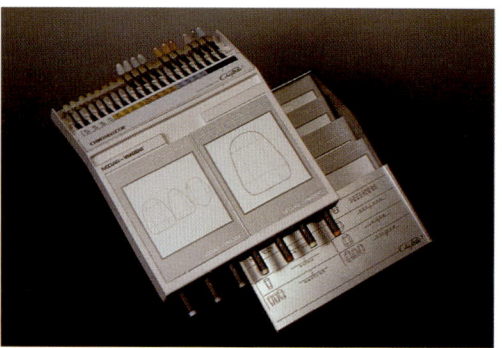

Fig 3-7 A revised Colour Communication system.

problems. More often than not, reliance is placed on unsatisfactory shade guides, and the hope that the technician will guess what the surgeon had in mind. Technicians frequently never see the patient or the actual tooth to be fixed. A step towards better colour matching and more natural aesthetics can be attempted by beginning with a compatible shade guide that reliably copies actual restoration colour.

Indirect resin shades are available in two linked shade guides, one for the intra-coronal inlay/onlay material, and the other for use with the extra-coronal crown, bridge and veneer material. Intra-coronal resin comes in seven basic shades, and these will cope with most clinical situations. Practitioners who have experience of using direct resin will notice that colour rendering is easy when intra-coronal restorations are placed. Light transmission through the tooth is not blocked by the resin material and some blending of colouration usually results. Extra-coronal resin needs a greater variety of shades in order to match natural teeth. One new guide contains twenty shades and these are based on 20 dentine shades, divided into five hues. The colours are based on dentine shades because it is dentine that gives the colour in teeth (Fig 3 - 6).

Extra-coronal resin (with the exception of laminate veneers) is designed to be fabricated with a metal supporting sub-structure. An opaquing system that also provides a strong bonding of the resin must be used, otherwise metal shine-through will mar the final appearance.

One overall system can be used, and this will permit accurate prescriptions to be given to the technician. By sticking to a system that encompasses all the restorative materials that may be blended in the restoration of a mouth, the dentist avoids the 'grey' area of 'mix and match' that frequently ends up in a strange mixture of different coloured teeth.

Careful attention to this aspect at the initial treatment planning stage can avert this and allow for the harmonious use of compatible materials to fix a selection of different problems in the same mouth. Throughout this book are examples where indirect resin is used in conjunction with light-cured resin to restore teeth with inlays, onlays, crown and bridge pontics and laminate veneers.

A comprehensive colour communication system (colour palette) is now available. This new system tackles the problem of effective colour communication using well researched principles to aid accurate colour control.

References

1   Croll, T.P. and Cavanaugh, R.R. (1986) Enamel colour modification by controlled hydrochloric acid-pumice surface abrasion. Quint. Int. 17:157.

2   Olin, P.S., Lehner, C.R. and Hilton, J.A. (1988) Enamel surface modification invitro using hydrochloric acid-pumice. Quint. Int. 19:733-736.

Suggested further reading
Muia, Paul J. (1985) The four dimensional tooth colour system. Quintessence.

Chapter 4

Onlay Modifications

The indirect resin system is well suited to the restoration and protection of tooth tissue and is able to serve as a long term restorative material.

Many teeth that require restoration also need cuspal protection, and these were traditionally repaired with metal (eg amalgam, gold) which is aesthetically lacking. The alternative treatment is the full coverage bonded crown. This is a good long term treatment but also entails further tooth cutting.

The advantages of cuspal coverage for protection against fracture are well accepted, and indirect resin can, and should be employed with this factor in mind.

Indirect resin material can be used to restore many teeth requiring cuspal protection as cuspal coverage onlays. Approximately 1.5 to 2 mm of tooth should be removed from the cusp in order to cover with indirect resin material. A flat non-bevelled margin needs to be made.

Every tooth that is prepared merits some thought being given to its long term durability and the preparation should therefore be modified, if necessary, by including one or more onlaid cusps in the design.

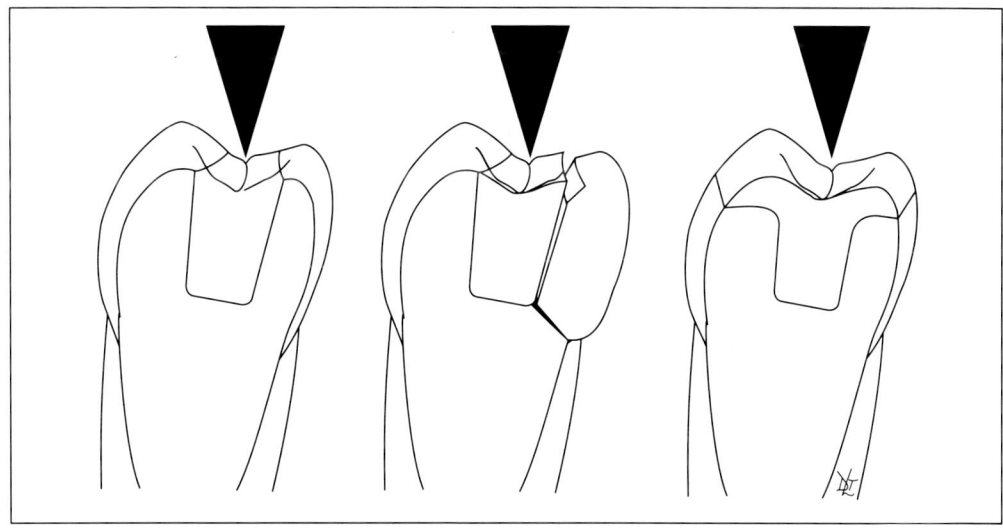

Fig 4-1 Cuspal Coverage for protection from fracture.

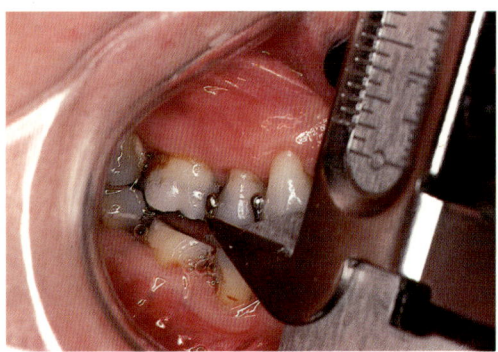

Fig 4-2 Adequate occlusal reduction is necessary.

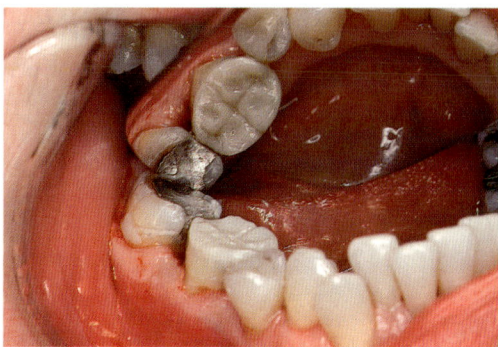

Fig 4-3 Mirror view of restored tooth.

The onlay process is a simple and effective way to improve the strength of many teeth. Figs 4-2 and 4-3 show how approximately 2 mm of occlusal reduction was made to allow a strong occlusal onlay to be provided on this (non-vital) tooth.

The final cavity design must also take into account other important factors such as the occlusal forces, the vitality of the tooth, and the shape of the remaining tooth structure.

A pre-operative assessment of the occlusal pattern will indicate whether or not special care will be needed to reduce the risk of fracture on the onlay. In general it is wiser to produce a non-interfering onlaid cusp in centric and eccentric functions.

The decision concerning the covering of cusps for protection should be determined after making a careful inspection of the remaining structure, and assessing the ability of the teeth to resist fracture. For example, a curved intact tooth wall is less likely to fracture than a straighter wall of the same thickness (Figs 4-4 and 4-5).

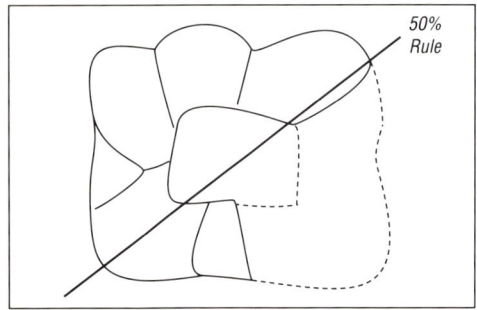

Fig 4-4 Inlay preparation. Where more than 50% of strong continuous tooth remains, an inlay preparation is acceptable.

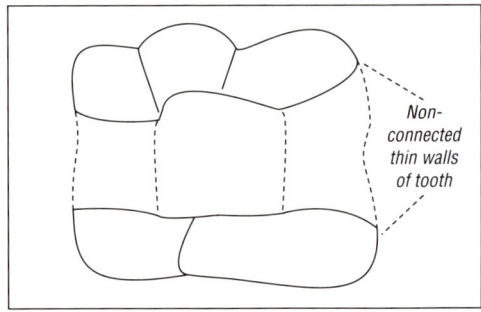

Fig 4-5 Onlay preparation. Where there are large MOD preparations with thin walls of tooth, full cuspal coverage is advisable.

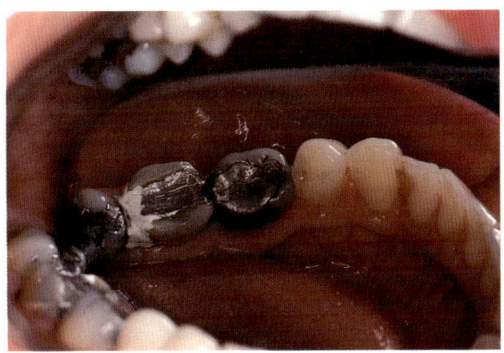

Fig 4-6 Both molars required re-restoration.

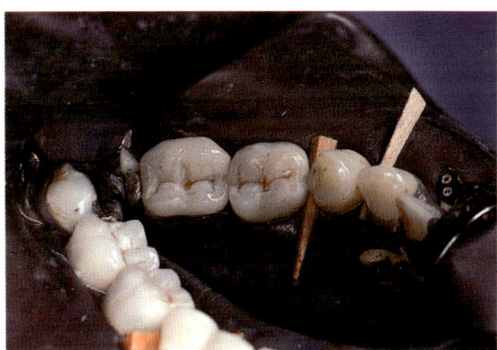

Fig 4-7 The aesthetic improvement is obvious.

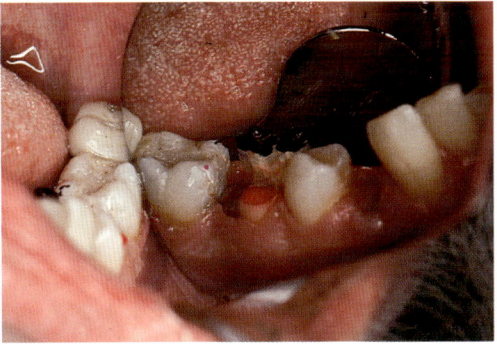

Fig 4-8 Red ink showing reduction of buccal cusp. Black ink showing lingual cusp to be covered.

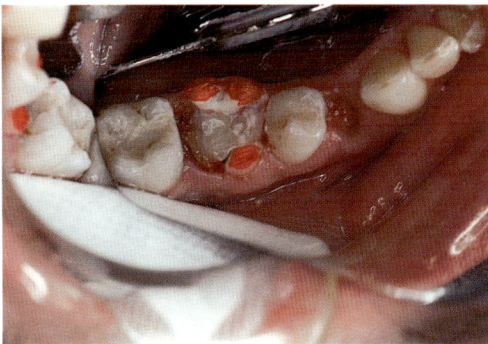

Fig 4-9 Red ink shows cusps which have been reduced.

Examples of both styles of preparation are illustrated in Figs 4-6 and 4-7, where the first and second lower molars required re-restoration.

In this patient an inlay style is adopted for one tooth whilst in the other an onlay version is chosen.

Teeth may not require cuspal reduction and protection where over 50% of the remaining wall of the tooth is substantial and intact, thus forming an arc. Cusp protection should be made where walls of tooth are straight and not continuous, and whenever the cusp is higher than it is wide.

The case shown in Figs 4-8 to 4-11 illustrate how indirect resin material should be used to restore a lower non-vital molar, where buccal and lingual tooth substance was not strong enough to resist possible fracture. Non-vital teeth should always be assessed for cuspal coverage.

After lining this tooth, both buccal and

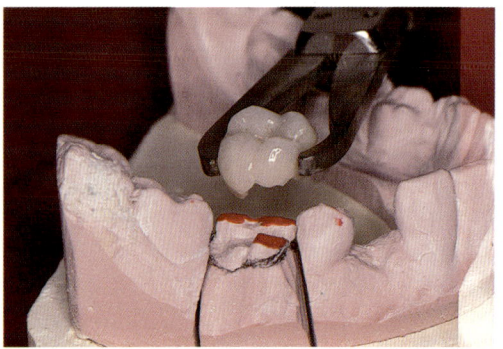

Fig 4-10 Onlay ready for insertion.

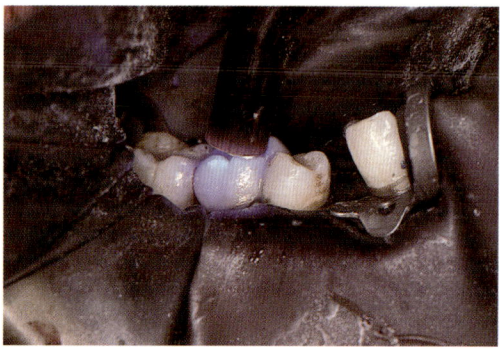

Fig 4-11 Onlay being attached using dual curing cement. Isolation with rubber dam is a great help when there are subgingival margins.

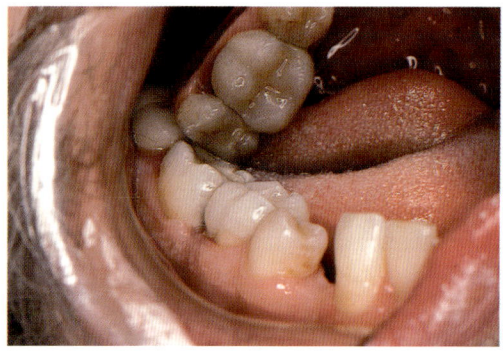

Fig 4.12 The completed restoration.

lingual cusps were reduced by 1.5 - 2 mm. In Fig 4 - 8 red ink shows where the buccal cusp has been reduced and black where the lingual cusp has not yet been protected. The resultant onlay resembled a gold cuspal-coverage onlay in design. Indirect resin is easier to make as no bevels are required; in fact, a marginal bevel is not a desirable finish: there should be a butt-joint.

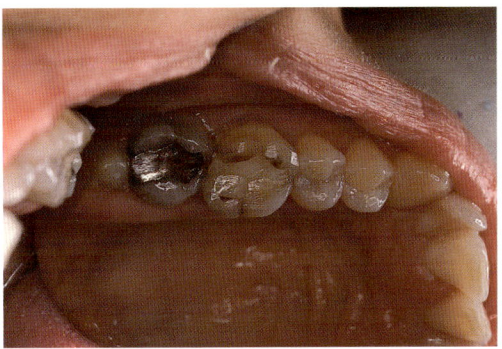

Fig 4-13 Direct resin failing due to recurrent caries.

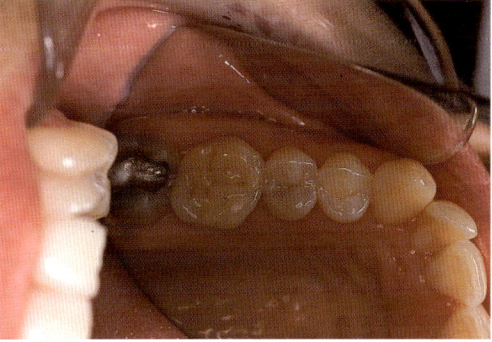

Fig 4-14 Partial cuspal coverage was appropriate.

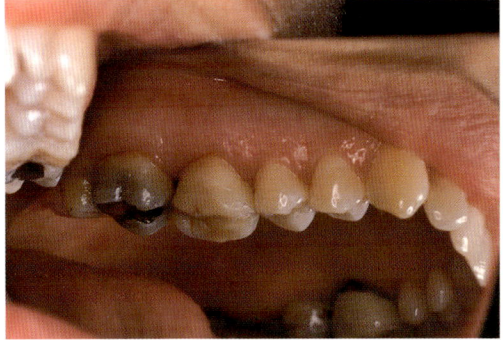

Fig 4-15 Final restored tooth was aesthetically superior to the adjacent second molar.

The onlay process is an integral part of the inlay/onlay system, and it can, and should, be incorporated into everyday inlay restorations. Teeth may deserve full coverage, partial coverage, or even protection of just one cuspal portion. The patient shown in Figs 4-13 to 4-15 wanted another aesthetic restoration in her first molar when she was informed that the existing direct composite filling was failing.

An assessment of the tooth structure remaining after removal of the old filling and recurrent caries revealed the need for partial cuspal coverage. It is hard to clinically detect that the buccal cusps have in fact been covered.

Yet another preparation variant can be considered when a non-vital molar (or premolar) is to be restored. The demands of modern endodontics frequently dictate large access cavities, and these teeth require restoration and cusp protection.

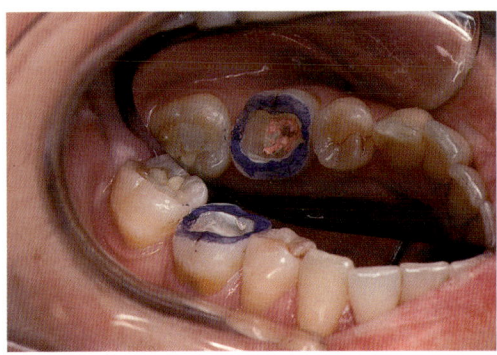

Fig 4-16 Non vital molar required restoration of the access cavity. Blue ink shows the vulnerable area to be protected.

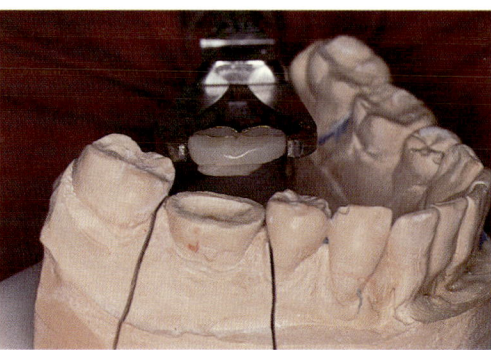

Fig 4-17 This simple preparation is easily accomplished.

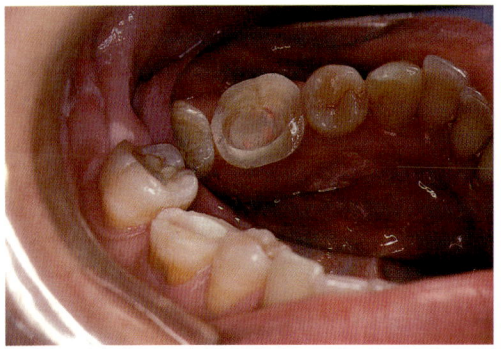

Fig 4-18 The entire occlusion is formed in the laboratory.

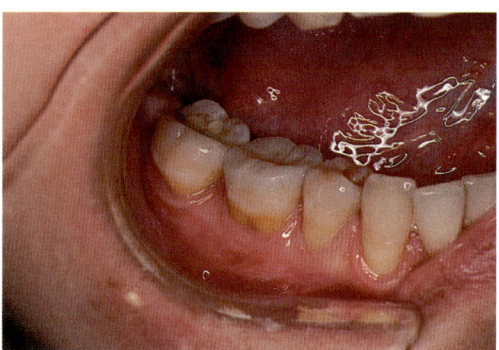

Fig 4-19 Finished restoration. Note that the excellent marginal tissues have not been encroached upon.

In the case of the patient shown in Figs 4-16 to 4-19 the large size of the access cavity and the pre-operative assessment of her occlusal habits suggested an onlay type of restoration. A simple reduction of 2 to 3mm together with an occlusal depression permitted a full coverage onlay to be fabricated.

In this way an aesthetically pleasing result was obtained without compromising the tooth. More examples of restoration of non-vital teeth are provided in Chapter 8.

Chapter 5

Intra-Coronal Modifications

Indirect resin can be considered for use wherever an aesthetic and functional restoration is required. It can replace the use of other traditional restorative materials in selected cases.

Indirect resin may be blended with traditional crown and bridgework. In the example shown in Figs 5-1 to 5-4 a fixed-moveable bridge design was chosen to restore the upper missing premolar. By substituting an indirect resin inlay for the traditional class 3 gold inlay in the canine the risk of metal 'shine-through' was avoided.

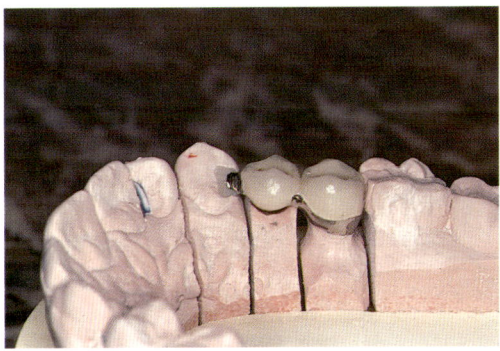

Fig 5-1 Modified fixed-moveable design incorporating indirect resin inlay.

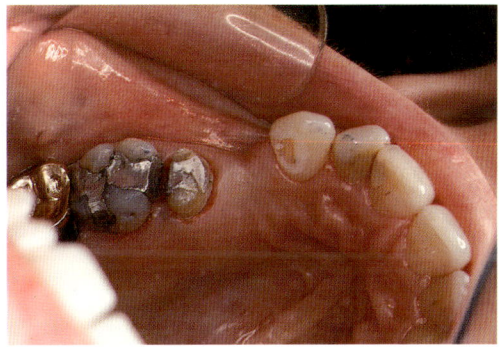

Fig 5-2 Inlay cavity etched prior to inlay cementation.

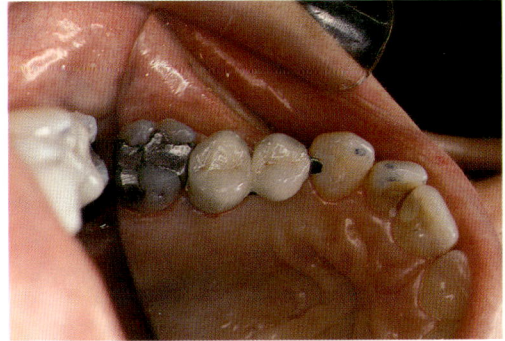

Fig 5-3 Mirror view of completed bridge.

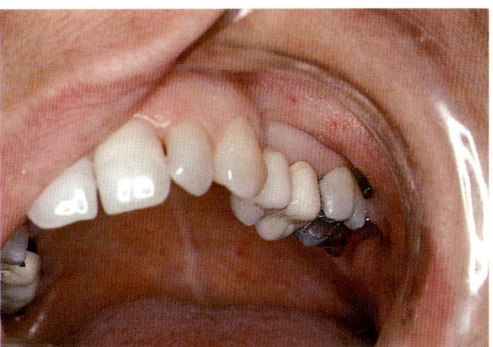

Fig 5-4 The completed bridge.

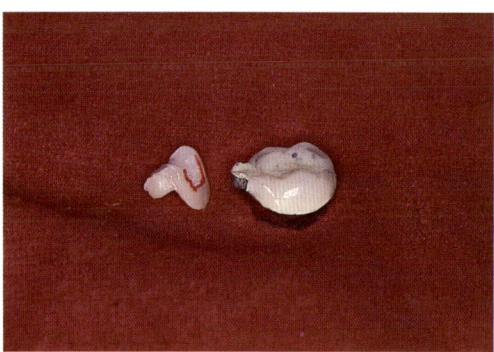

Fig 5-5 Laboratory prepared rest seat marked with red ink.

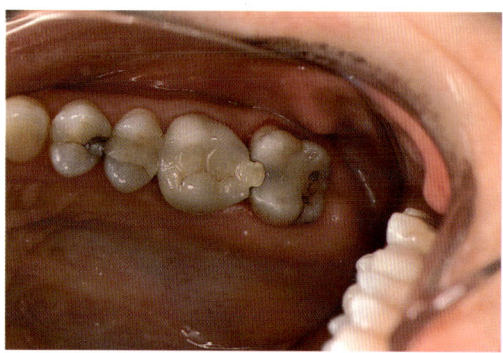

Fig 5-6 The completed case.

The aesthetic superiority of using this material is evident from the photographs. It may also be argued that the acid-etched bonded margin is superior to the cement seal of a gold inlay, thus reducing another weak link in the restoration.

Figs 5-5 and 5-6 show indirect resin used to restore a second molar tooth, providing a rest-seat for an occlusal rest from the first molar crown. This rest eliminated a food-packing problem between the teeth.

Indirect resin inlays are also suitable for larger restorations where a superior aesthetic result is required. The case shown in Figs 5-7 to 5-9 illustrates a common problem — that of a vital pre-molar with a fractured palatal cusp. Teeth like these frequently had large occlusal fillings and one or more cusps eventually fractured. This alternative treatment plan shows how the range of use of indirect resin may be extended. A pinned inlay was made for this patient.

Two parallel pin holes were drilled in the palatal position. Williams pins (plastic burn-out pins) were inserted in the holes and, after coating the pins with adhesive, an impression was taken. The pins, now captured in the impression were used as burn-outs and cast in gold.

The resultant inlay was cemented into position. The same Dual-cure resin cement was used to bond the inlay and pins; only the enamel margins were acid-etched. The patient was delighted with her restored tooth.

Caution

Indirect resin is primarily designed as a non-pin retained material. The essential feature is the bonding resin cement which chemically attaches to the resin and bonds to the etched enamel margin. Nevertheless, the experienced clinician and technician can extend the range of uses, as in this case. An alternative method could utilise a dentine adhesive as the retentive aid in place of pins.

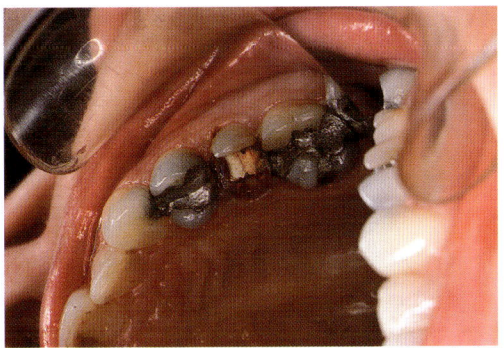

Fig 5-7 A common problem: Vital tooth with only buccal cusp remaining.

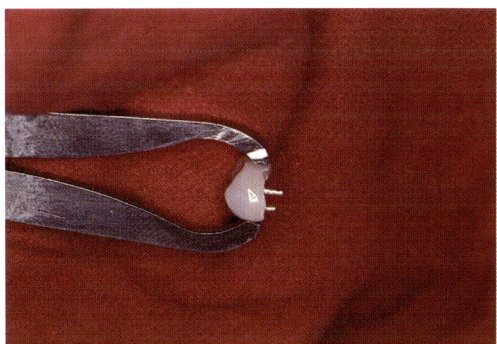

Fig 5-8 Pin retained onlay.

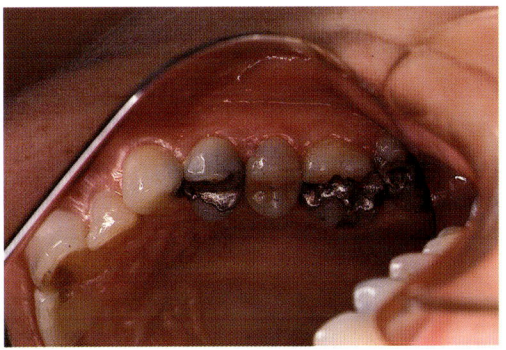

Fig 5-9 The completed case.

Incisal repairs

It is common for adults as well as children to need treatment for chipped and fractured incisor teeth and light cured resin fillings continue to offer a quick way of restoring these teeth. However, the well known consequences of wear and staining eventually cause these restorations to fail. They may serve well enough for the younger patient, who expects to have the work done again at a later time, though adults deserve a more durable job. Porcelain pieces have been successfully used in the repair of incisal fractures in cases where a chip or class four fracture was insufficiently severe to warrant a labial laminate veneer or, indeed, a full coverage crown.

The advent of indirect resin inlays has largely replaced the need for porcelain 'pieces' and pinned composite fillings. Direct resin is most commonly used for these cases and a microfill composite will probably exhibit the least wear. Nevertheless indirect resin can also be used whenever the need to minimise wear is important. An indirect resin class four restoration could be expected to wear at the same rate as natural tooth substance, as long as there are no adverse occlusal factors.

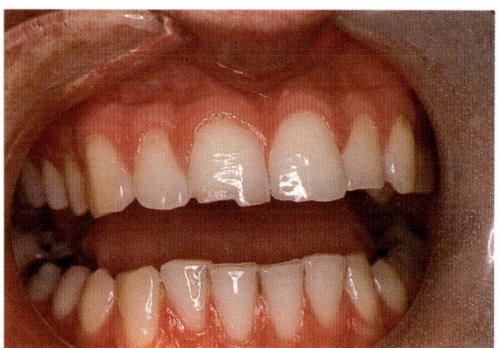

Fig 5-10 Before treatment: Direct resin would be an alternative material.

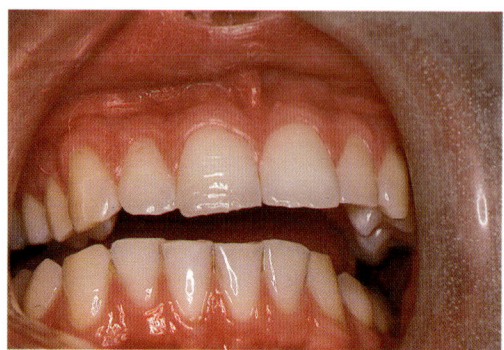

Fig 5-11 After cementation of Inlay.

The young adult shown in Figs 5-10 and 5-11 required the restoration of a chipped upper incisor in which the fracture was entirely within the enamel. The preparation conformed to the requirements of the acid-etched retained restoration. The one millimetre rule was observed — (Jordan: *Esthetic Composite Bonding*). It has been demonstrated that a 1 mm etched margin provides sufficient retention for a composite restoration, without the need for additional retentive measures, such as undercuts or pins.

The enamel adjacent to the fracture was prepared to a thick chamfer margin, approx. 1 mm past the fractured margin on both the labial and palatal surfaces, and an impression made.

Indirect resin should not be used in thin sections and a feather margin should be avoided. A substantial clearly defined preparation is required. The technician made an indirect resin restoration which was cemented at the second appointment.

Lower incisors also present with fractures and these are more difficult to restore with direct light-cured resin. Indirect resin material is a suitable material for dealing with these teeth: it is strong enough to last and excellent aesthetic restorations can be made. The special preparation is done as shown in Fig 5-12.

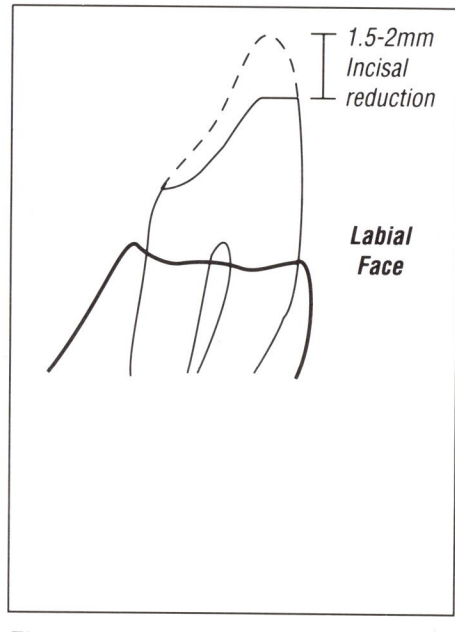

1.5-2mm Incisal reduction

Labial Face

Fig 5-12 Onlay preparation for vital lower incisor.

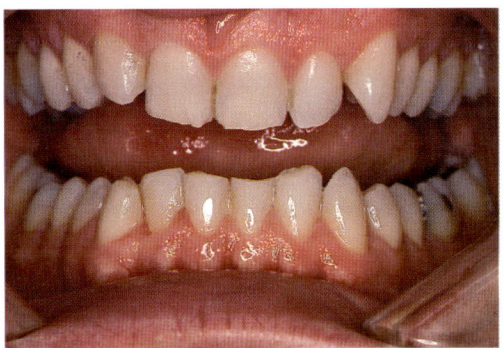

Fig 5-13   Fractured lower incisors.

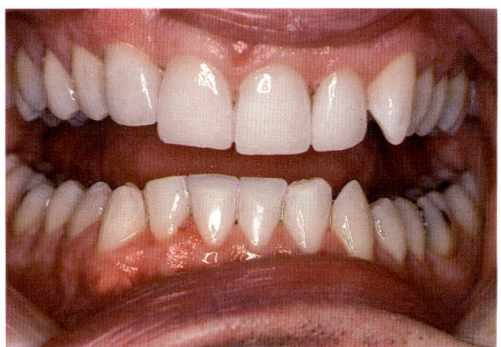

Fig 5-14   After placement of two incisor onlays. (Note the upper incisors were veneered.)

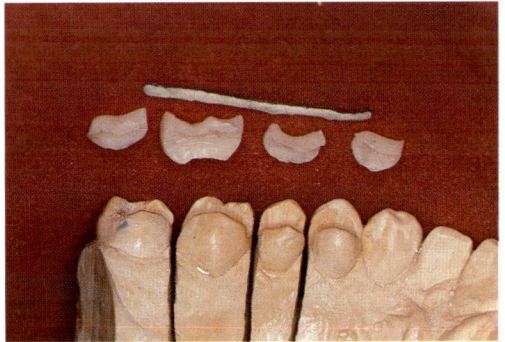

Fig 5-15   Separate inlays and a fitted cast metal bar were made.

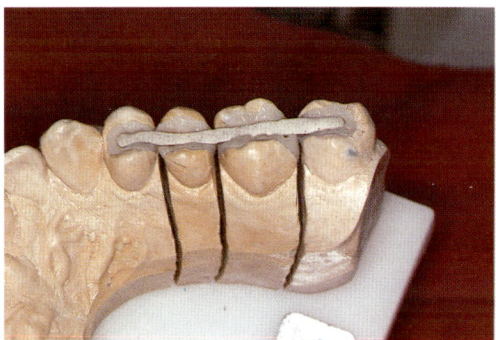

Fig 5-16   The metal bar was covered with a ceramic opaque.

Indirect resin material can also be used in most situations where light-cured resins are indicated, for example in closure of interdental spacing (diastemata), and in modification of tooth contour for aesthetic reasons or to create undercuts for removable prostheses.

Splinting

Secure intra-coronal splinting can easily be accomplished with linked indirect resin inlays. Several loose premolars

and molars can be fastened together in a simple two-visit procedure.

On the first visit the MOD channels are prepared; in many instances occlusal restorations are already present and these may be replaced without further loss of tooth tissue. An impression is taken and the teeth temporised. Light cured resin (Fermit) is convenient and quick to use. The technician will make separate inlays as indirect resin inlays cannot be fabricated in combined units. He will then cut an occlusal channel and make a cast or wrought metal support to run passively in the channel. By countersinking the structure beneath the occlusal plane the metal can be concealed with light cured resin.

On the second visit the inlays are first tried in the mouth, to ensure proper fitting. Upon cementation the inlays are firstly inserted and the metal frame tried in to check that it lies passively in the channel. Tooth movement between appointments, particularly in periodontally compromised teeth, may mean that some adjustment is necessary. The resin of the inlay may easily be cut away with an air rotor. The metal is cemented into position with a light-cured resin of medium body. Wedges should be inserted interdentally to prevent flow of the resin.

Caution

Whilst secure linked inlays can provide excellent splinting, careful appraisal of occlusal patterns needs to be made at the planning stage. Where a large differential in occlusal forces is noted, the potential for debonding should be acknowledged. These teeth should all be covered with linked full coverage gold onlays.

Chapter 6

Crown and Bridgework

The indirect resin system is well-suited for use in standard crown and bridge-work. Generally speaking the indications for using this material are the same as for acrylic resin and to a large extent as for fused porcelain as well. Indirect resin material can be supported by precious, semi-precious and non-precious alloys. It adheres well to these metals and a well proven laboratory technique should be followed. A well tried and tested method of attaching the resin to the metal utilising retention beads ensures a strong attachment to the sub-structure and metal shine-through is eliminated by the application of an effective opaquing agent. A chemical linking agent (Spectra-Link) provides additional retention.

The same principles concerning comparative wear rates govern the choice of the occlusal surface in these cases. Indirect resin material may be used as the entire pontic or crown exterior when a wear rate comparable to natural tooth substance is acceptable. A recent study[1] demonstrated that indirect resin was satisfactory as a substitute for porcelain when used as a buccal facing on posterior crowns. In fact, crowns may also be made with entire buccal and occlusal coverage whenever the loss of approximately 7 microns per year is not significant. This particular study used facings of laboratory cured resin that extended halfway down the buccal cusp towards the central fossa. In this way gold occlusals preserved the holding contacts.

In areas where aesthetics is of prime importance, such as the mandibular premolar area, this design can be altered to allow full occlusal coverage with the resin. Two methods of marginal design are appropriate for indirect resin bonded onto gold (or metal) crowns.

Metal margin

A bevelled shoulder design permits a gold collar to be made and this may be attached with a luting cement and then burnished. This excellent method (Fig 6-1) is suitable whenever the display of a gold collar is not a problem.

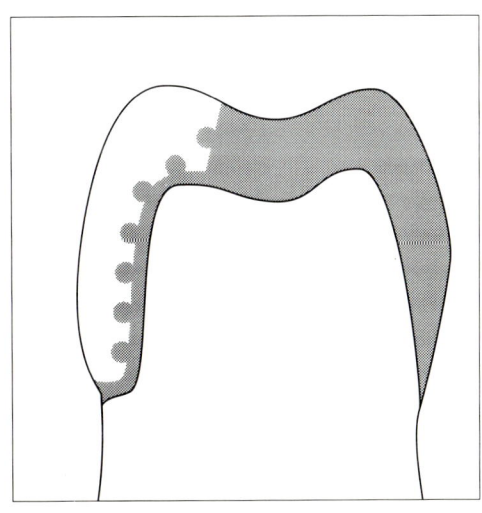

Fig 6-1 Metal margin design.

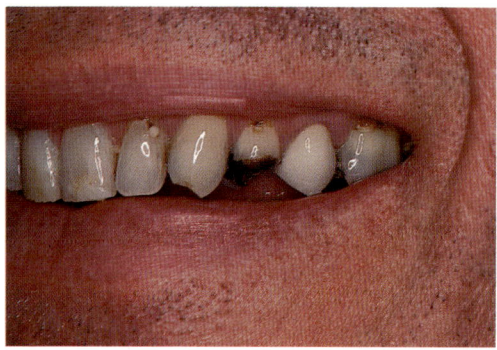

Fig 6-2 Upper first premolar (vital) requires a full coverage crown.

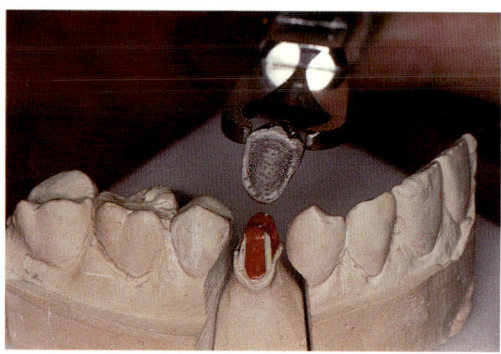

Fig 6-3 The metal design before indirect resin is applied. Note parallel slots to improve retention of the crown.

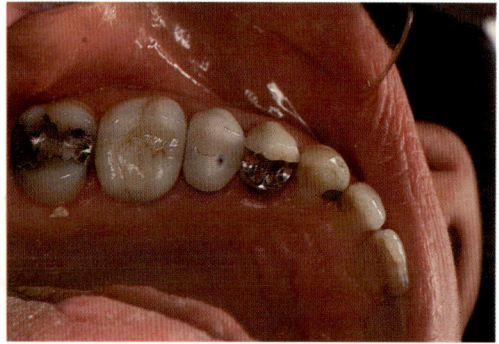

Fig 6-4 Occlusal view of fitted crown; note the existing porcelain bonded to metal crown on the second premolar tooth.

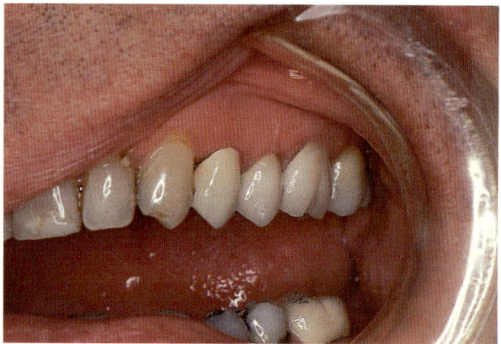

Fig 6-5 The completed crown; the gold collar is not obtrusive, and the smile line of this patient conceals all the margins.

The patient shown in Figs 6-2 to 6-5 required a full coverage restoration on his first premolar tooth. The pre-operative assessment included a check on the position of his smile line. The margins of the premolar teeth were covered by his lips so it was possible to employ this method without compromising on the final aesthetic result.

A gold sub-structure was fabricated, and the resin facing extended halfway down the palatal slope of the buccal cusp. Micro-retentive beads were cast onto the facing area to enhance retention and the chemical Spectra-Link process employed in the laboratory.

Resin bonded margin

A more aesthetically pleasing result can be obtained by utilising the special quality of indirect resin: that of compatibility with resin cements. A chamfer-shoulder margin design, which is easy to produce, allows the technician to make a butt-fit facing, that extends past the

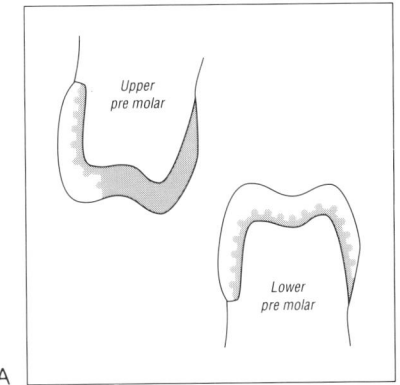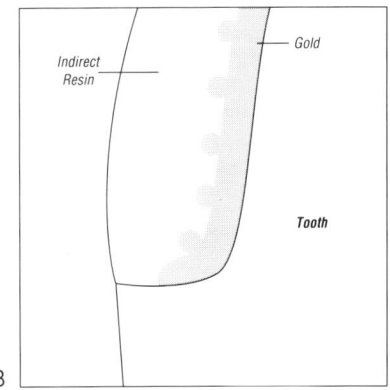

A

B

Fig 6-6 Resin margin design (A) with enlargement of margin area (B).

gold casting (Fig 6-6). Unlike porcelain, there is less difficulty in obtaining a butt-fit because there is no firing shrinkage.

Not only is the gold margin eliminated, but the tooth margin can be primed with a dentine bonding agent (such as Syntac). The margin can then be polished to give a very smooth join indeed. Where all the margins are on sound enamel, etching will allow a very secure bond.

Traditional principles of tooth preparation should be adhered to, and sufficient tooth reduction made to allow for a metal thickness of at least 0.5 mm and additional space of 1 to 1.5 mm for the resin.

For example, the facial surface of an incisor tooth requires reduction in two planes: one parallel with the path of insertion, and a second parallel with the incisal two-thirds of the tooth (Fig 6-7). A definite shoulder facially and a chamfer palatally should also be made. Indirect resin material requires satisfactory metal support. Indirect resin material is suitable for bridgework as well as for single crowns. The material should be

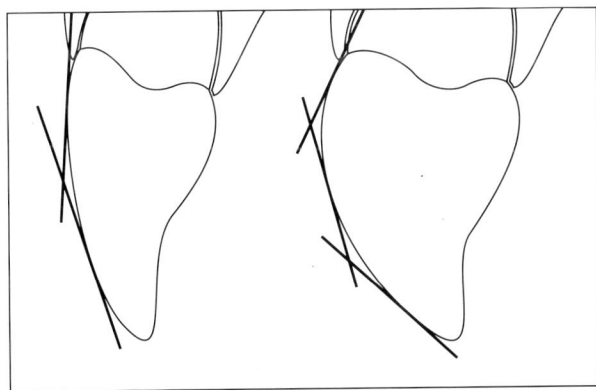

Fig 6-7 The canine (cuspid) tooth, above right, needs reduction in three planes. With acknowledgements to Cassidy, McLaughlin and Grey.

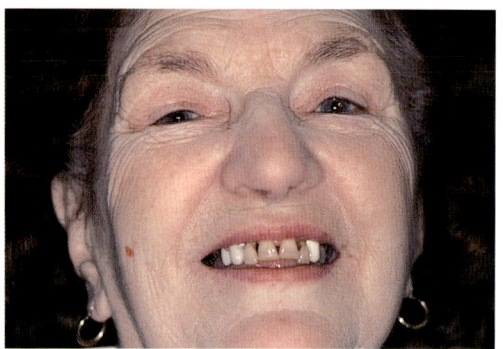

Fig 6-8   Patient before treatment.

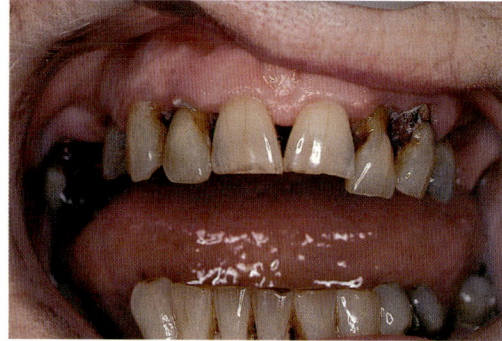

Fig 6-9   Intra oral view of patient in Fig 6-8.

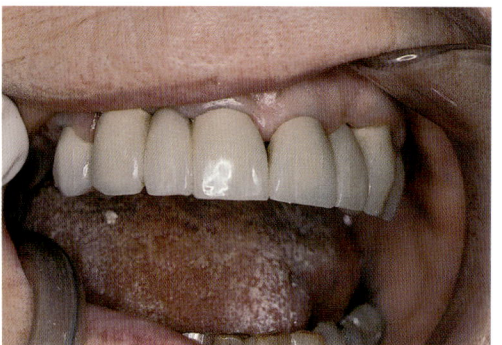

Fig 6-10   The completed case.

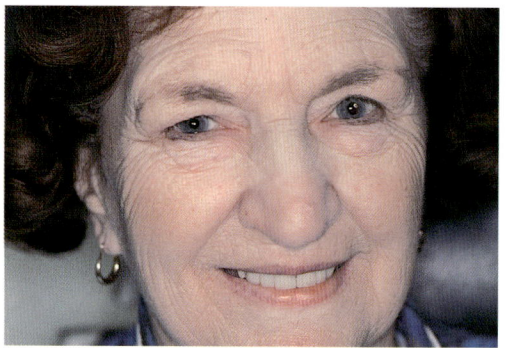

Fig 6-11   A delighted patient smiles happily.

supported by a cast metal sub-structure. The laboratory process will ensure a firm bond to the metal (see technical section).

The elderly lady shown in Figs 6 - 8 to 6 - 11 needed extraction of both periodontally-involved lateral incisors. Unlike the patient in Figs 6 - 4 to 6 - 7, this woman's smile line revealed all the margins of her upper incisors, and so the resin-bonded design was chosen.

Two indirect resin bonded to gold 3-unit bridges were fitted as an immediate replacement following extraction of the teeth, and the bridgework attached with a soft access cement.

This allows for adjustment to the pontic contours, if necessary, after the healing period. In this way subtle changes in the form of the pontic can be made permitting a more natural pontic/tissue margin to be established. Self-cure or light-cure resin can easily be added to indirect resin.

An advantage of indirect resin is that additions and repairs may be made. Complete polymerisation occurs during the curing and as a result no free radicals remain for bonding. This is not an obstacle to bonding as a special bond enhancer (Special Bond II) has been developed for this situation.

The surface to be bonded should first be roughened and the bonding enhancer applied and light cured. It is then possible to add resin directly, and this will form a secure attachment. This case illustrates how the flexibility inherent in this material permits subtle modifications to be carried out if necessary.

The patient was delighted with her new smile, and this treatment has certainly improved the quality of her life.

Occlusal design for full coverage restorations

Fig 6-12 illustrates suggested lower arch and upper arch designs for indirect resin bonded to metal crowns.

The physical properties of both materials need to be borne in mind, and the best blend of appearance and structural integrity chosen. Lower incisors and premolars can be faced in resin, the incisal edge covered and extended onto the lingual aspect. In these teeth aesthetics takes priority over strength, and the occlusal forces are generally less than in the molar region. Molar design should be followed as shown: the buccal cusp faced in resin which extends halfway down the lingual slope of the buccal cusp.

A similar design is followed when constructing upper crowns. Upper incisors should have the entire labial face in resin, including the incisal tip. The palatal surface can then be formed in metal as this important occlusal area determines the anterior guidance. Care needs to be taken with upper canines. Occlusions may either be canine (cuspid) guided or of the group function type. In both instances the occlusion should be assessed before commencing, as in all operative dentistry. Metal palatal surfaces should be used, with the entire incisal tips covered with resin.

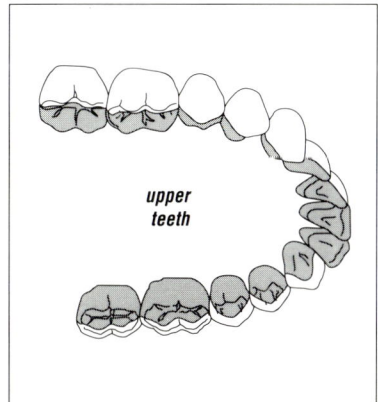
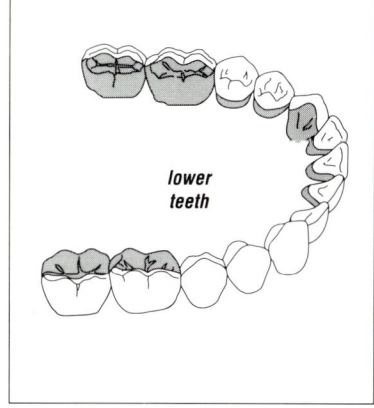

upper teeth

lower teeth

Fig 6-12 Occlusal design for full coverage restorations.

References

1   O'Neal, S.J., Mueninghoff, L. and Leinfelder. (1990)
    Clinical evaluation of Isosit-N as a coronal veneer.
    Univ. Alabama at Birmingham.

Chapter 7

Laminate Veneers

Labial (laminate) veneers are now well established as an effective way of restoring aesthetics. A variety of indications include: covering stained and discoloured teeth; repairing chipped and unsightly restored teeth; correcting mild irregularities, and alteration of contour. The restorative dentist who wishes to preserve what remains of his patients' natural tooth substance cannot afford to neglect this treatment modality.[1] [2] [3] [4]

Laminate veneers have been formed from self-curing resins directly in the mouth and also from pre-formed facings. Indirect veneers may be made from both porcelain and indirect resin material.

Indirect resin veneers and porcelain veneers have essentially the same range of clinical applications. Although glazed porcelain cannot be bettered for a natural enamel-like appearance, the indirect system also provides excellent aesthetic results.

Etching and silanization of the veneer is not necessary. Indirect composites utilise the chemical bonding resin to secure a bond to both enamel and the veneer fitting surface.

The ease with which resin veneers may be accomplished opens up opportunities that were more difficult to treat with porcelain. For instance the treatment of younger patients where the demanding clinical technique can be a handicap. Resin veneers can be altered and repolished in situ, and this feature is very useful when subtle changes to the emergence angles are desirable. The polished surface of indirect resin is comparable to that of glazed porcelain, and is tolerated as well by the gingival tissues. These qualities of resin veneers probably make them the material of choice when covering non-vital teeth: subgingival margins are essential to completely mask all discoloured tooth substance.

A further advantage of selecting a system that permits matching of light cure and indirect resins is obvious when a patient, such as the case illustrated in Figs 7-1 and 7-2, requires a blend of restorative work that includes both labial veneers and direct composite resin fillings.

The young man was given a satisfactory improvement to his stained and irregular front teeth by simply instituting oral hygiene; subsequently providing him with two laminate veneers to correct the instanding central incisors; and re-filling the lateral incisors with the appropriate shade of direct light-cured composite, chosen by the same shade guide. The patient was delighted with his new front teeth and is now motivated to keep his teeth cleaner.

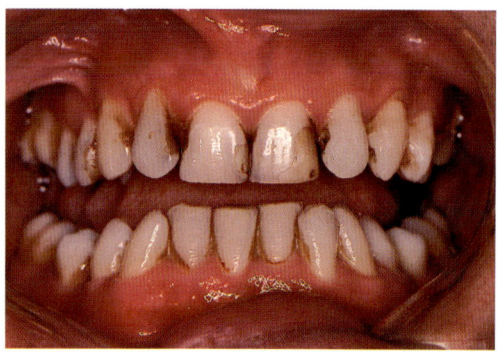

Fig 7-1 Before treatment. The patient requested aesthetic improvement.

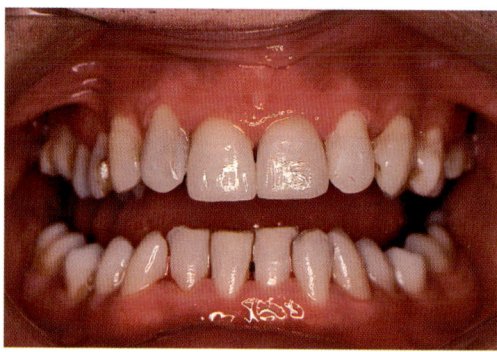

Fig 7-2 Only two veneers were necessary.

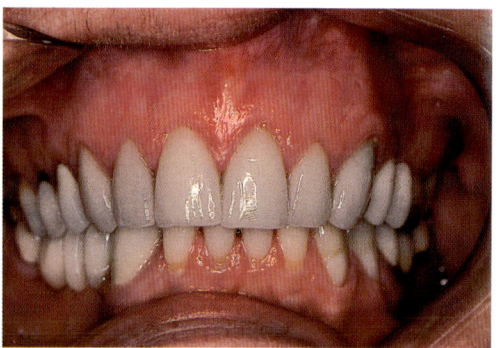

Fig 7-3 Excellent tissue health around veneers.

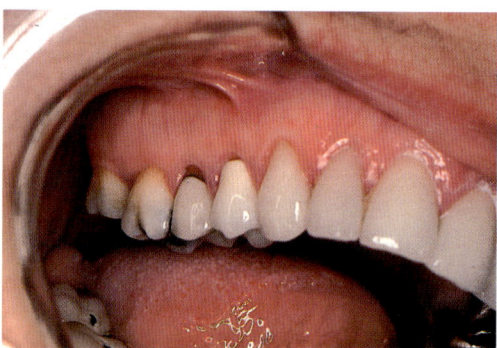

Fig 7-4 The same patient showing recession buccally to crowns on both premolar teeth.

Periodontal aspects

Laboratory processed laminate veneers merit serious consideration as a viable alternative to full coverage crowns. One hallmark of laminate veneers is the excellent tissue health and lack of gingival inflammation after placement. This fact has caused a re-think about the association of gingival inflammation and recession around full crowns. Both indirect resin material and porcelain veneers are capable of achieving a fine margin. Full crowns can also be well fitted, although certain undesirable sequelae can occur. Delayed recession leading to exposed margins often happens with time, but this does not seem to occur with veneers to the same extent. More research is needed to back up this clinical impression.

Recent studies (including a three year report by Gordon and Rella Christensen and a five year study by Ronald Jordan of the University of Ontario) are tending to reinforce the view that laminate veneers are associated with excellent marginal tissue health. One factor that may explain this stems from the differences in tooth preparation between full crowns and veneers. Only in the full crown preparation does the bur pass through the embrasure. This delicate interdental part of the periodontal attachment is vulnerable to trauma.

Fig 7-5 shows shows the difference in height between the buccal gingivae and the interdental tissue.

Injury to the interdental tissues easily leads to localised recession — ie apical migration of the attachment. This in itself would not become visually apparent were it not for the genetic programming that ensures a constant relation in form between the periodontal attachment and the marginal bone. A loss of height interdentally can lead to a loss of height buccally, and this may explain the phenomenon so often seen around crowns. This phenomenon may be related to the concept of 'Biologic Width'. Recession following periodontal injury is only one of the undesirable consequences that may occur: an alternative reaction is pocket formation with or without bone loss.

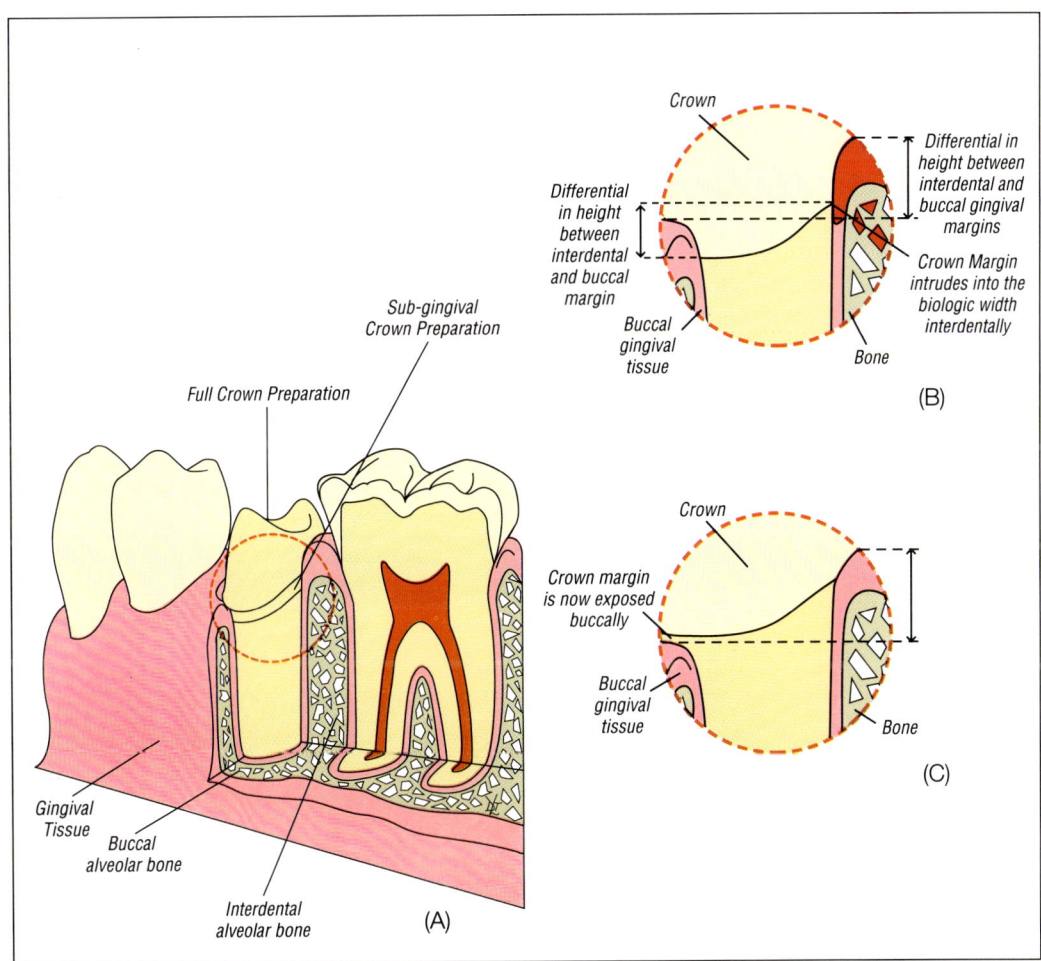

Fig 7.5 (A) A diagrammatic section of an interdentally over-intrusive crown preparation. (B) An enlargement of the crown margin area. (C) Gum recession is one possible consequence of the overpreparation.

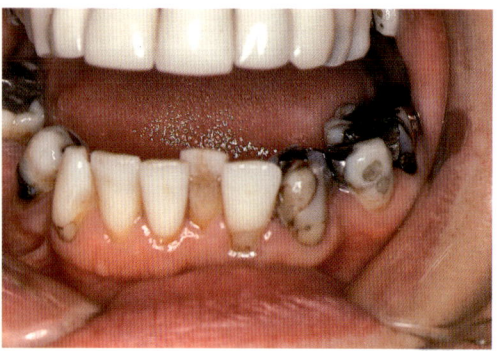

Fig 7-6 Before treatment. In-standing lower incisor was unsightly.

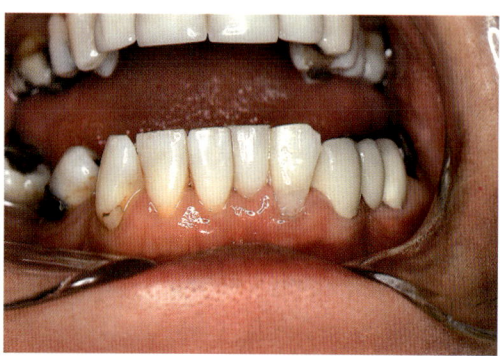

Fig 7-7 Following treatment. One veneer was fitted, and a three unit bridge placed to restore the side teeth.

It is obviously very useful to be able to predict whether or not gingival recession is likely to affect the aesthetic outcome of restorative dentistry. In fact in clinical practice it is often possible to gauge which kind of effect is more likely in a particular patient by a pre-operative assessment of the 'tissue type'. It has been observed that most people tend to fall into one of two 'tissue types': those with thick periodontal tissues, and those with thin tissues (although this distinction is not always clearcut). The periodontal consequences of damage or disease to thick tissues tends towards pocket formation, whereas those with thin tissues are more prone to gingival recession.

The wise practitioner should be very careful before embarking upon aesthetic restorative dentistry on patients with thin tissues. Full metal bonded to ceramic or resin crowns can, and do, provide excellent aesthetics and give strong restorations. Laminate veneers not only provide excellent aesthetics but also lessen the risk of periodontal damage. In fact sub-gingival preparation is unnecessary because the tissues do not seem to recede. Veneers may be finished at, or just below the gingival margin with confidence. Laminate veneers can also be provided in combination with other treatments to improve aesthetics.

In the case shown in Figs 7-6 and 7-7, an instanding incisor was fitted with a single veneer in order to improve alignment. The patient was not willing to undergo orthodontic correction of her crowded teeth.

Caution

As with every restorative procedure, badly finished laminate veneers have the potential for causing periodontal damage. All bonding cement must carefully be removed following placement and the margins polished to a high lustre. It has been shown that the slight increase in bulk of a tooth following attachment of a veneer does not, in fact, contribute to gingival inflammation. With the clinical evidence of so many satisfactory laminate veneers, the theory that over-contouring teeth leads to periodontal problems can finally be discounted.

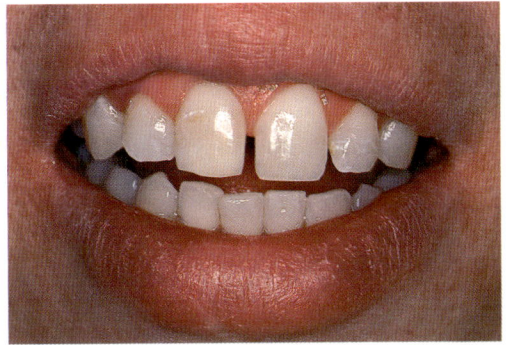

Fig 7-8 Patient requested gap to be closed.

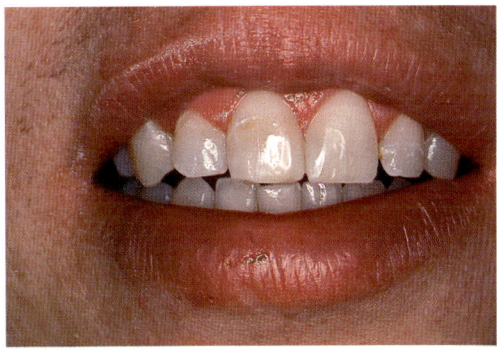

Fig 7-9 Direct resin used on these otherwise intact teeth.

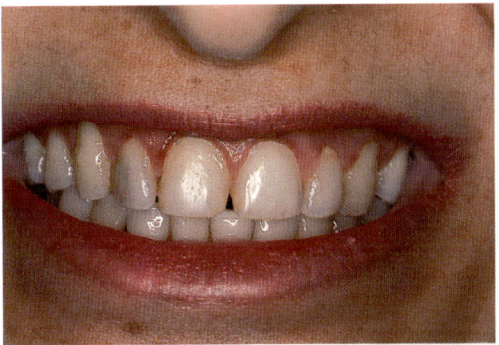

Fig 7-10 Before treatment.

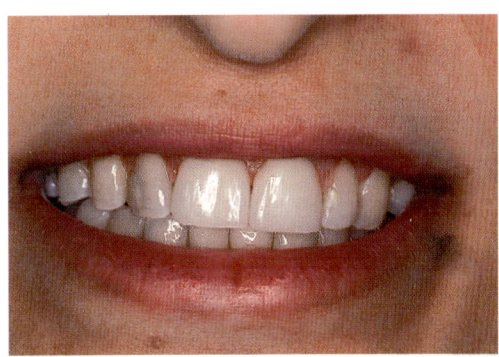

Fig 7-11 Two laminate veneers enabled teeth to be elongated, as a compensatory measure to restore pleasing proportions.

Diastema closure

Spaces between front teeth are disliked by some people and these gaps can usually be closed quite simply if not too great in width. The two most conservative methods, aside from restoring with full crowns, are with direct and indirect resins. There are clear differences in the indications for each type, as is illustrated in the next two clinical examples.

Unblemished and intact teeth are candidates for direct resin additions, as in the example shown in Figs 7-8 and 7-9.

Teeth that have been filled, or teeth with imperfect enamel should be ven-

eered. This also permits complete control of the morphology of the labial faces, as in the case illustrated in Figs 7-10 and 7-11 where the teeth were elongated to improve the aesthetics.

Caution

A careful pre-operative assessment of the patients' occlusion is essential in these types of cases. Veneers can be used to lengthen clinical crowns only where the incisal guidance does not interfere with the new veneers, or else veneer fracture is invited. The appearance of increased length can often be created by other means, as in the next clinical example.

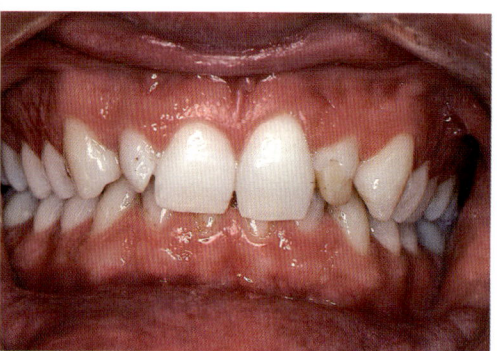

Fig 7-12 Before treatment.

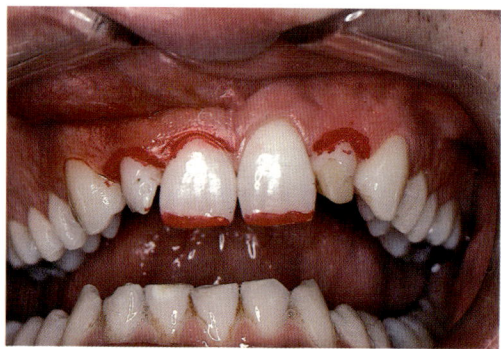

Fig 7-13 Following a pre-surgical assessment of the various forms of altered eruption this case was able to be corrected by simple resection. Red dye shows where both tooth tissue and gingival tissue are to be removed.

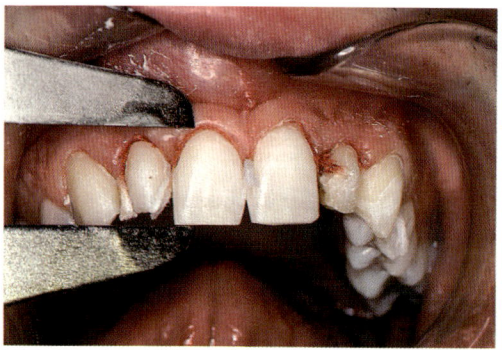

Fig 7-14 The length of the incisors has been made equal by a blend of surgery and incisal reduction.

Clinical procedures for producing laminate veneers

A young man of 21 years (Fig 7-12 to 7-22) was so self-conscious about his dental appearance that he was reluctant to smile in public. He requested treatment to improve his smile. Evaluation of his case revealed a mild class two, division two irregularity with, in addition, the phenomenon of altered passive eruption, leading to shorter than normal clinical crowns.[5]

Caution

The various types of altered eruption need to be studied before any attempt at treatment is considered.

Six weeks after the application of electrosurgery to correct soft tissues the six upper teeth were prefaced for veneers. Careful measurements were taken to ensure that the technician had the correct space in order to produce well aligned veneers.

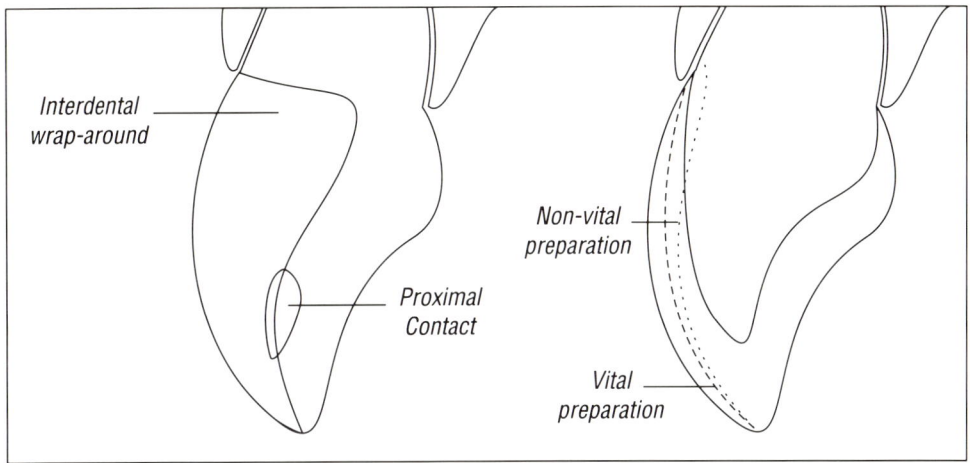

Interdental
wrap-around

Non-vital
preparation

Proximal
Contact

Vital
preparation

Fig 7-15 A cross section and a side view of tooth preparation for an indirect resin veneer.

The steps required to achieve indirect resin veneers are explained here, using this patient as an example.

First clinical appointment
The patient should be consulted and an appropriate shade chosen from the shade guide, taking into account certain factors detailed below.

The teeth to be prepared may have dried and moisture loss can affect colouration, causing them to become lighter and more opaque. This should be explained to the patient and an allowance made. The difference in colour between incisors and canines should also be explained. Although it is technically possible to attach veneers to unprepared teeth, some degree of surface preparation almost always permits a better result to be achieved. One suitable bur kit is the Komet, and this includes two-grit burs that simultaneously roughen the labial enamel and create a finer gingival margin. A chamfer

margin is to be preferred and is easier to work to than a knife-edge. The gingival margin needs to be extended only to the edge of the gingival sulcus, or just below it. Deep sub-gingival preparations are not required, or even desirable. (One exception to this is when a non-vital tooth needs a veneer. Non-vital tooth colour is usually different from the adjacent vital tooth, or it gradually becomes so. It is therefore important to cover all visible supra-gingival tooth substance, both labially and interdentally.) Approximately .5 to .75 mm of labial enamel should be removed to make room for the veneer. This is variable, for some teeth require additional reduction in order to reduce a mal-alignment. Patients will often be more comfortable with a local anaesthetic in place during this procedure.

The next step is to prepare the embrasure area. The important element in this process is to avoid cutting through the contact area between teeth, therefore avoiding cutting the gingival tissues. All vital teeth should be cut with copious water cooling, and the teeth kept wet with damp pads until the impression stage. The incisal edge of the preparation can be finished at the incisal edge of the tooth and does not need to cover it. In this way the veneer will be the same length as the original tooth.

In this respect the standard preparation differs from the preparation to receive a porcelain veneer, when incisal coverage is generally used. Incisal coverage for the purpose of elongation can nevertheless be adopted, subject to the provisos already mentioned. A clear finish line should be made, so the technician can see the extent of each veneer. Sharp internal angles should be avoided. The completed veneer preparation should have sufficient 'wrap around' to cover all the visible buccal tooth, but not extend through the contacts. Polishing is not advisable as it reduces the roughness and hence the surface area for bonding. A fine braided retraction cord is then carefully inserted and left in place for a few minutes.

Impressions

A full-arch impression is the best way to aid the fabrication of veneers as the technician needs to have some idea of the arrangement of the dental arch and the morphology of the teeth. A material that allows for at least two models to be poured should be used. Temporization is not normally required. Should temporary veneers be requested, these can quickly be formed using direct resin, which can be adapted over each tooth and light cured into position. The polymerisation shrinkage alone will retain these unetched veneers until the next appointment.

Second clinical appointment

The veneers should have been made according to detailed instructions to the technician, and returned ready for fitting. All characterization should already have been incorporated into the veneers.

The teeth surfaces should be cleaned with pumice and a thin abrasive strip passed through the contacts to remove debris from the borders of the preparations. This important stage should not be omitted, otherwise marginal contamination will cause an unsightly discolouration around the completed veneers. The veneers can then be tried in individually, and then all together to evaluate the fit. Glycerine should be dabbed onto the tooth surface, otherwise an air space would alter the colouration. If a veneer seems too light or too dark at this stage, it may not necessarily be unsuitable. The final colour of a veneer may be influenced by the choice of bonding resin shade. A kit containing a selection of resins should be available, and these can be tried in place without curing the resin. The unpolymerised cement can then be removed with acetone.

Caution

Light, and self curing resins may change in colour after curing. This takes place in two stages. The first stage occurs during curing, and depending upon the make can be either a lightening or a darkening. The second stage occurs in the days that follow initial curing and this is usually a slight darkening. The operator should be aware of the characteristics of the make of resin that is used. Veneers are very delicate until attached to teeth, and must be handled with great care in order to avoid breakage. They should not be altered either, except when contacts are tight and prevent correct placement.

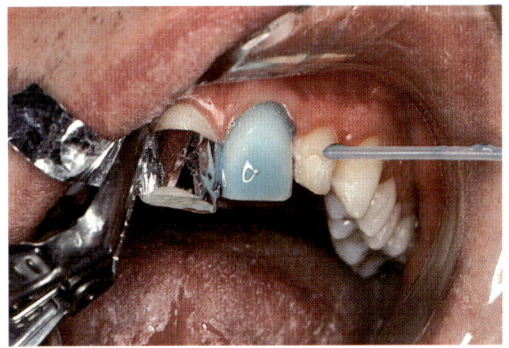

Fig 7-16 The central incisor is etched.

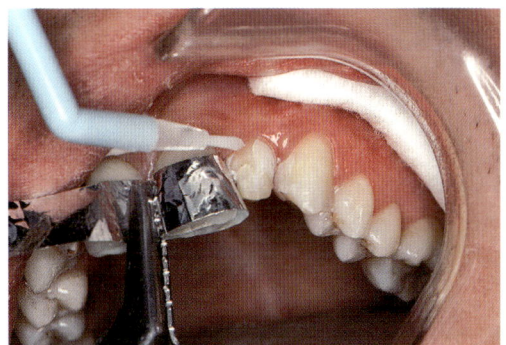

Fig 7-17 Application of dentine adhesive to etched lateral incisor.

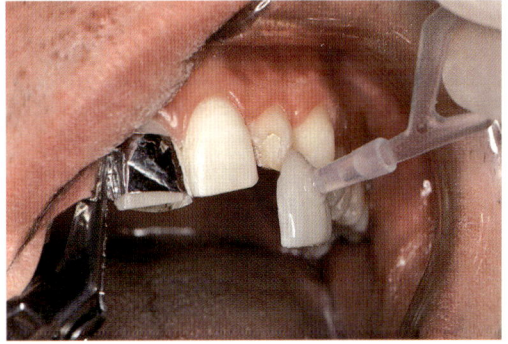

Fig 7-18 Veneers should be handled with great care.

The Colour coupling effect discussed in Chapter 3 can then be assessed and a trial attachment of various resin cement colours (eg Heliolink). This effect is not apparent without a cement medium between the veneer and the tooth.

The Colour coupling effect is determined by the underlying dentine colour. The use of colour modification by resin cements should be considered as secondary 'fine tuning'.

The tooth should then be etched for 15 to 30 seconds with 37% phosphoric acid. Gels are easier to control. Each tooth should be isolated from its neighbour, and thin foil (such as 'space blanket') introduced between each tooth to accomplish this without creating spacing.

The acid must be thoroughly washed off with oil-free water spray, and a warm air draught wafted over the frosty enamel to properly dry it. A hair-dryer is a useful piece of equipment.

Indirect resin veneers are easier to attach than porcelain veneers. Each veneer is coated with a layer of 'Special Bond II' resin, and this light-curing bonding agent is allowed to dry for 20 seconds and then light cured for 40 seconds.

Should labial enamel be deficient, a dentine bonding agent such as Syntac

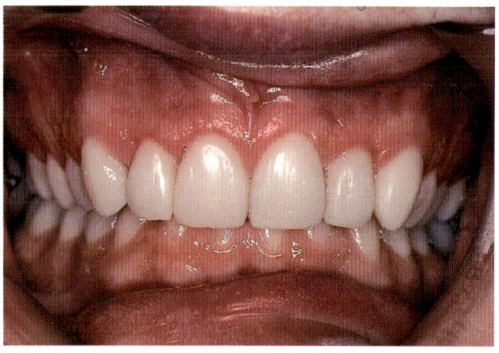
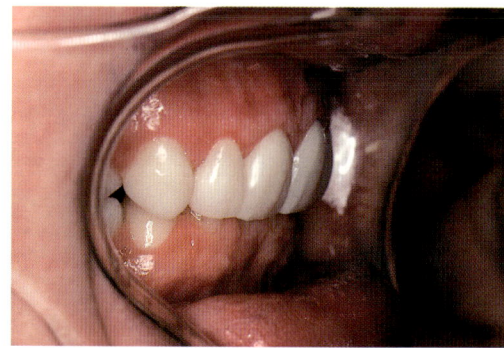
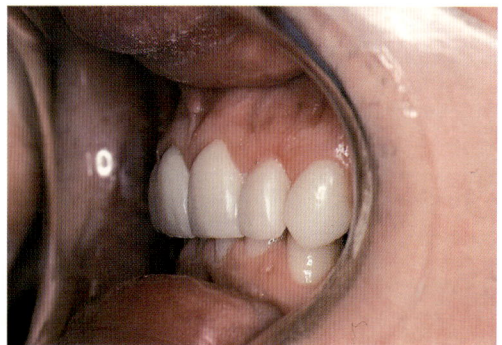
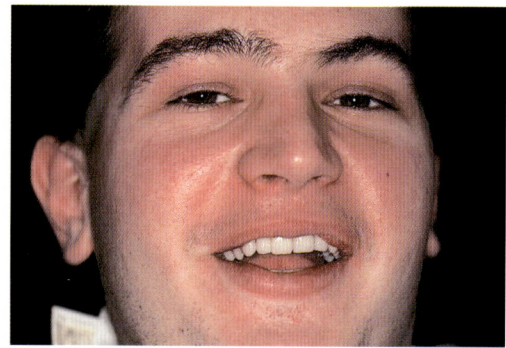

Figs 7-19 to 7-22   The final result and a smiling, happy patient.

should be used to enhance bonding. The desired shade of resin bonding material is then mixed and the veneer gently eased into position with a soft 'jiggling' motion. Excess resin can be removed after a 10 second cure, before it hardens completely. Fig 17 shows how a dentine adhesive was applied to the lateral incisor where enamel was deficient.

It is important to completely cure the resin with light over a period of at least 90 seconds, beginning with the incisal tip. Following polymerisation, the margins can be finished and polished taking great care to remove all residual resin. The interdental areas can be polished with graded strips, and the gingival areas with polishing cones.

As can be seen this patient was transformed and he left the surgery with greatly increased self-confidence.

Dentine adhesion
Indirect resin is primarily designed as an acid-etched enamel retained system. Only enamel may satisfactorily be etched, to provide resin-tag attachment for the bonding process. Whilst sufficient retention is generally provided for Intra-coronal inlays/onlays utilising etched enamel, extra-coronal restorations may need additional adhesion when enamel is deficient.

Laminate veneers may nevertheless be attached to teeth that, after preparation, lack a complete enamel face. Improved dental adhesives such as 'Syntac', may be used to advantage to improve the bond to the veneer. Dentine adhesive also prevents post-operative sensitivy that can occur following placement of resin.

Uses of opaquing resins

Many teeth exhibit staining which the patient would like corrected. These teeth can frequently be treated by using an opaquing resin before placing veneers. Opaquing resins are compatible with indirect resin material and form a secure bond. However, a better form of treatment would be to lighten the teeth with a bleaching technique before veneering, as the colour coupling effect of the veneering process will permit better aesthetics.[6]

Any opaquing medium placed between teeth and veneer will obstruct light transmission and give a rather 'dead' lifeless appearance. Teeth that are so dark as to present a problem should be restored with full coverage crowns.

Non-vital teeth

The treatment of non-vital teeth with veneers is covered in Chapter 8.

References

1   Pincus, C.R. (1938) Building mouth personality. J. S. Calif. Dent. Ass. 14:125-129.
2   Christensen, G.C. (1985) Veneering of teeth: the state of the art. Dent. Clin. N. Am. 29:373-391.
3   Fleming, J.E., Bayne, S.D., Spence, P. and Taes, C.G. (1984) Month clinical evaluation of laminate veneers. J. Dent. Res. 63:1082.
4   Calamia, J.R. (1988) Alpha Omegan vol. 81, winter, pp. 48-51.
5   Coslet, J.G., Vanarsdall, R.C. and Weinsgold, A. (1977) Diagnosis and classification of delayed eruption of the dento-gingival junction in the adult Alpha Omegan.
6   Stean, Howard. Unpublished report.

Suggested further reading

Garber, Goldstein and Feinman. (1988) Porcelain laminate veneers. Quintessence.

Chapter 8

Restoration of Endodontically Treated Teeth

Modern concepts relating to the restoration of endodontically treated teeth are shifting from dogmatic treatment plans to a newer realization that individual assessment of each case may, in many instances, point to better, more conservative methods. (See Table 8-1.)

Two important changes in dealing with non-vital teeth concern the aesthetic consequences of the endodontic treatment itself and the role of post reinforcement. Several studies[1] [2] [3] allude to the fact that a post crown is not always the strongest way to restore a non-vital tooth. Posts may not impart greater strength to a tooth, and may in fact weaken it and create the danger of root fracture.[4] The rationale for inserting a post is shifting from 'reinforcement' to a rather different concept; that of providing retention of the core and the preservation of the maximum remaining tooth structure. An all too common problem is that of root fracture associated with a post crown; such teeth need to be extracted and so share the fate of so many other endodontically treated teeth.

Several factors contribute to problems in restoring root-filled teeth. The brittle un-nourished dentine loses its natural colouration and is frequently stained by endodontic chemicals as well as the degradation products of pulp tissue. Much of the crown is often missing due to caries, fracture, and access cavities,

and for these reasons a post-retained crown is most often advocated.

However, when each tooth is properly assessed it will be seen that a 'blanket' approach should not always be taken.[5] [6] The new approach to the restoration of endodontically treated teeth is illustrated in Fig 8-1 to 8-3.

An upper molar of a young woman was root-filled and required restoring in an aesthetic manner. A passively cemented post was used to help retain a deep lining of glass-ionomer cement. A direct resin could have been used but would have been difficult to shape well. This lining is ostensibly the 'core' of the tooth. It is important to understand that this lining forms a bond with the inlay and therefore allows for stress to be distributed throughout the root and tooth. Glass-ionomer cement is one useful material in this respect, due to its ability to be etch-bonded to resin such as indirect inlay material. The choice of inlay design was governed by the amount of tooth substance remaining. Intact buccal and mesial walls, that were substantial, enabled a modified Class Two inlay to be successfully made.

More frequently it is desirable to cover cusps in order to protect them from fracturing and the onlay process is generally advisable.

The fundamental principle of preserving what remains holds in restoring

TABLE 8-1

Alternative Restorative Treatment for Non-Vital Teeth

Tooth Position	Treatment	Comments
Upper incisor (instanding)	Consider single laminate veneer	A post may not be needed where sufficient dentine remains. A modified prep. is essential to extend the margin sub-gingivally and to wrap around inter-dentally in order to cover all discoloured tooth
Multiple incisors	Consider laminate veneers	Any tooth with large access cavity and/or inadequate coronal dentine may need a post retained core
Lower incisor	Consider inlay/onlay to restore access cavity plus incisal edge	A simple procedure which gives a good aesthetic result provided the labial face of the tooth is unblemished
Upper and lower premolars	Consider heat/pressure cured resin crown with integral post	Standard plan of post crown with porcelain is always to be considered, but a variety of complications may suggest alternative approaches
Lower molars	Consider inlay/onlay	Aesthetic demands are more stringent in the lower arch *Caution:* Although heat/pressure cure wears at a similar rate to natural tooth it may sometimes be necessary to resort to gold occlusal in order to preserve occlusal stability
Upper molars	Consider inlay/onlay	Aesthetic considerations become less important towards the back of the mouth
		Smile factors must be evaluated before deciding the best option. The smile in repose and in normal and extreme positions needs to be assessed in consultation with the patient

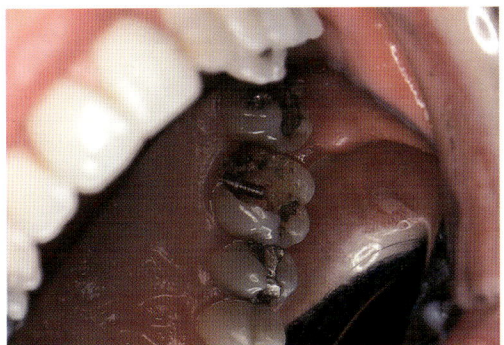

Fig 8-1 Pre-formed post inserted in palatal root canal.

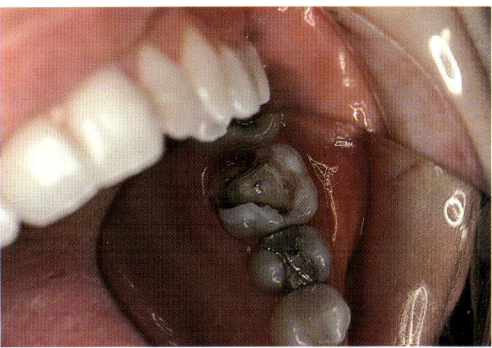

Fig 8-2 Lining placed in position.

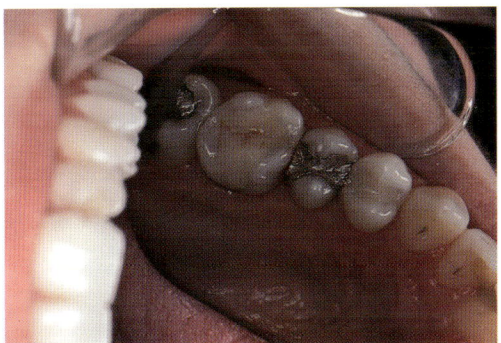

Fig 8-3 The restoration completed.

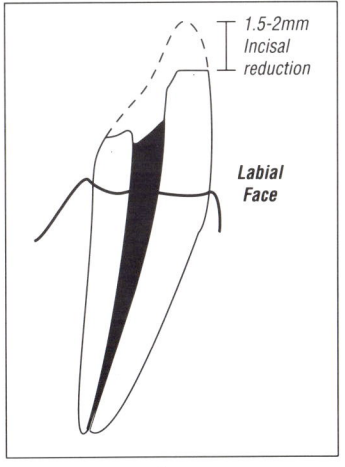

1.5-2mm Incisal reduction

Labial Face

Fig 8-4 Diagram of onlay preparation for an endodontically treated incisor.

endodontically treated teeth as in vital teeth. It is not easy to re-create the beauty of natural teeth and that is a good reason for thinking again before drilling away the labial face of a tooth in order to restore it. Indirect resin material offers another way of restoring teeth without the unnecessary removal of tooth substance.

The lower incisor tooth can be difficult to restore following endodontics. Loss of tooth substance often dictates provision of a post crown. An alternative approach, when the enamel face is in good condition, is to prepare the tooth for an onlay employing the special modification to fill the access cavity (Fig 8-4).

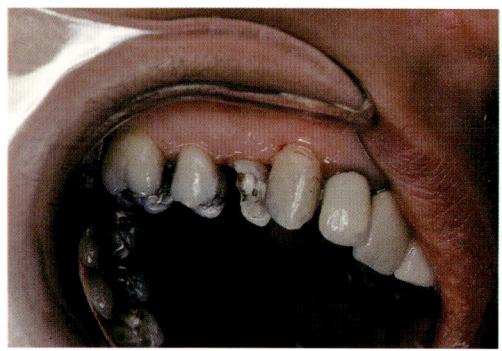

Fig 8-5 Tooth with loss of buccal wall requires post crown.

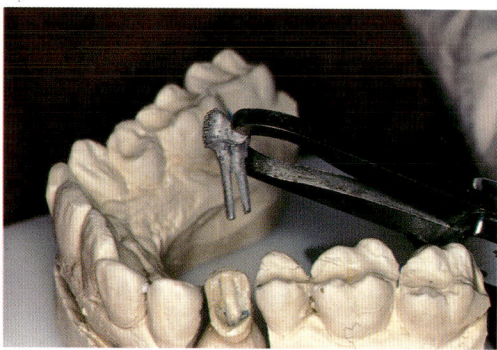

Fig 8-6 Post can be tried in to check fit.

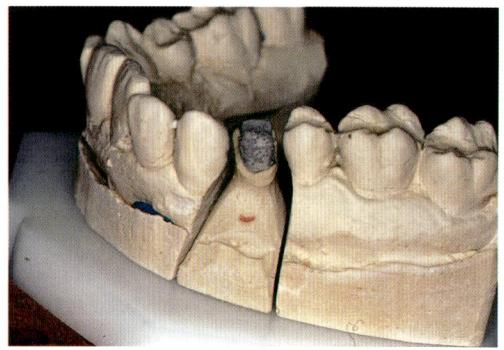

Fig 8-7 Metal is finished 1mm short of all margins.

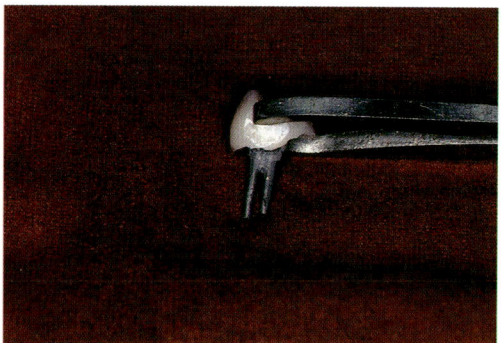

Fig 8-8 Crown ready for placement. The same laboratory process as crownwork is employed to mask all metal and prevent shine-through.

Resin bonded post crown techniques

Cases where a post crown is required are usually when there has been loss of the natural buccal enamel wall. Indirect resin crowns with posts can be made for these teeth. One advantage of indirect resin is that it bonds to etched tooth material using resin cement. This feature can be used to advantage in a modification of the post crown in which a resin margin rather than a metal margin is created.

A young woman attended the practice with a badly carious upper first premolar which required endodontic therapy (Figs 8-5 to 8-11). All factors were evaluated, and it was decided to restore the tooth in the least destructive way. An indirect resin bonded to gold crown was made, incorporating an integral post and core, and with a palatal supra-gingival margin on enamel.

One criticism of integral crowns is lack of good fit. This may be due to a variety of laboratory factors, including metal and porcelain shrinkage. Selecting an indirect material negates

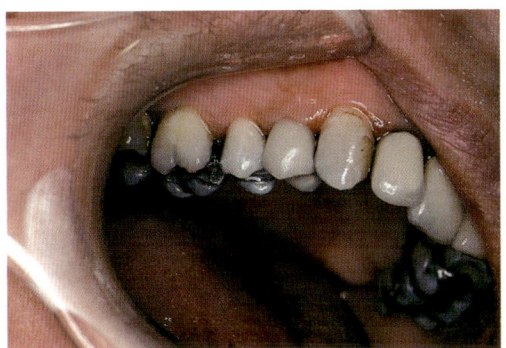

Fig 8-9 Completed crown.

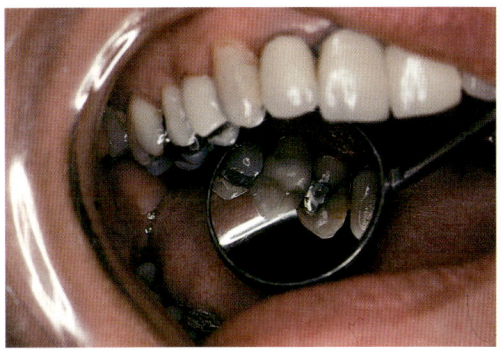

Fig 8-10 The palatal margin is undetectable by probing.

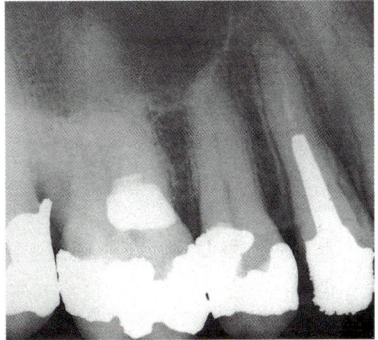

Fig 8-11 Radiograph of completed case.

this as a compatible bonding resin fills and seals the margins, which are secured on clean etched enamel. This more conservative preparation, which need not be entirely sub-gingival, retains the maximum of the remaining tooth. Recent research[7] [8] [9] [10] [11] [12] [13] with a resin retained posts is encouraging.[00] A passively fitted post with a loose fit reduces the chances of stresses that contribute to root fracture. It has been shown that resin cement can produce a strong bond in these cases.

Post crowns may be formed in a variety of ways. This method is simple and conservative to tooth structure. The patient was grateful that virtually all the remaining original tooth had been preserved.

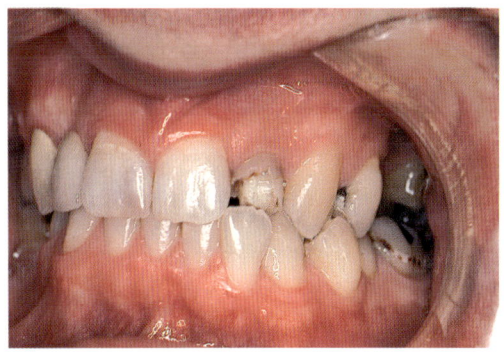

Fig 8-12 Non vital tooth requiring a post crown.

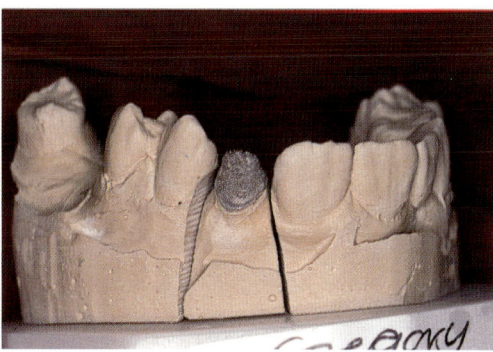

Fig 8-13 Cast post and core on model.

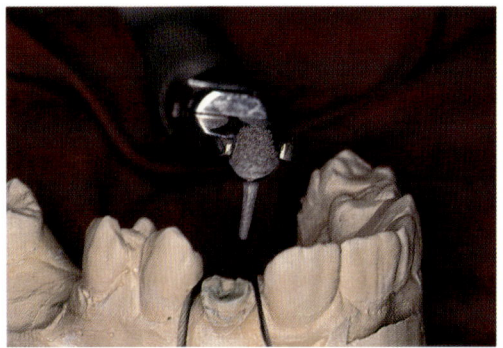

Fig 8-14 Note the micro-retentive beads.

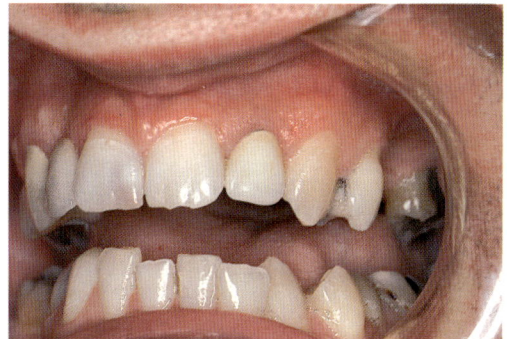

Fig 8-15 Completed case — metal margin not obvious.

Conventional post crown techniques

Indirect resin post crowns are well suited to accepted methods of post-crown construction. In the example shown in Figs 8-12 to 8-15 an integral gold post and core was made and the gold extended entirely around the margin onto sound tooth substance. This 'Ferrule Effect' has been researched and shown to decrease the danger of root fractures. Resin cement is not essential for this type of crown, and the operator may select the cement of his/her choice.

Laminate veneers for non-vital teeth

Laminate veneers can successfully mask mild discolouration that occurs in many root-filled teeth. A preliminary assessment will be necessary to discover whether the clinical crowns are likely to resist fracture. Teeth with strong enough crowns ie those with sufficient coronal dentine remaining, can be veneered and indirect resin material is probably the material of choice in these cases, as a certain quality of resin enables well adapted veneers to be formed when the use of porcelain would present difficulties: it can be reshaped and repolished following attachment.

Veneers cannot be well formed unless some tooth preparation is carried out. This step is even more important when discoloured teeth need re-facing. The modified preparation needs to extend sub-gingivally and inter-proximally. Otherwise the result will be marred by a dark line around each veneer.

Indirect resin can be attached to the tooth and delicate alterations made to the emergence angles until the appearance is entirely satisfactory. This step would be harder to accomplish with porcelain. Dark stains can be opaqued out with the resin available for this purpose.

Bleaching of dark teeth preparatory to veneering offers a better chance of good aesthetics, and this can be done in the surgery, or at home with one of the bleaching systems now generally available.

Combined bleaching/veneering techniques are quickly becoming an accepted treatment modality.

References

1 Guzy, G.E. and Nicholls, J.I. (1979) In vitro comparison of endodontically treated teeth with and without post reinforcement. J. Prosthet. Dent. 42:39.

2 Mattison, G.D. (1982) Photoelastic stress analysis of cast gold endodontic posts. J. Prosthet. Dent. 48:407.

3 Travert, K.C., Caputo, A.A. and Abou-Rass, M. (1978) Tooth fracture: a comparison of endodontic and restorative treatments. J. Endodont. 4:341.

4 Sorensen, J.A. and Martinoff, J.T. (1984a) Intracoronal reinforcement and coronal coverage. J. Prosthet. Dent. 51:780.

5 Trabert, K.C. and Cooney, J.P. (1984) The endodontically treated tooth: restorative concepts and techniques. Dent. Clin. North Am. 28:923.

6 Eissman, H.F. and Radke, R.A. (1987) Postendodontic restoration. From: Cohen, S. and Burns, R.C. Pathways of the pulp. Pub. C.V. Mosby.

7 Assif, D. and Ferber, A. (1982) Retention of dowels using a composite resin. J. Prosthet. Dent. 48:292.

8 Assif, D. and Bleicher, S. (1986) Retention of serrated endodontic posts with a composite luting agent. J. Prosthet. Dent. 56:689.

9 Goldman, M., DeVitre, R., White, R. and Nathanson, D. (1984a) An S.E.M. study of posts cemented with an unfilled resin. J. Dent. Res. 63:1003.

10 Ashayeri, N. and Nathanson, D. (1988) In vitro retention of different post systems. 66:344.

11 Goldman, J., DeVere, R. and Tenca, J.P. (1984) A fresh look at posts and cores in multirooted teeth. Compendium 0:71.

12 Nicholls, J.I. (1988) Rebuilding the treated tooth. J. Calif. Dent. Ass. 16:34.

13 Sorensen, J.A. (1988) Preservation of tooth structure. J. Calif. Dent. Ass. 16:15.

Suggested further reading

Shillingburg, Hobo and Whitsett. (1982) Preparation of extensively damaged teeth. Pp.150-155, Fundamentals of fixed prosthodontics. Pub. Quintessence.

Chapter 9

Indirect Resin Materials
in Adhesive Bridgework

Reliable adhesive bridgework is a further development that permits aesthetic fixed prosthetics to be carried out with a minimum of intervention. There are numerous indications for adhesive bridges and the indirect resin system may be selected as an alternative to the fused porcelain pontic with the advantage of easier aesthetics.[1] [2] [3]

One criticism of the adhesive (Maryland) bridge has been the display of metal rests and wings. This may not necessarily be a problem with upper bridges, and the initial case assessment

will show up the potential problem before the bridge is made.

In this example (Fig 9-1) a young man required the restoration of a missing first upper premolar. Note how an inlay was used to refill a small mesial occlusal cavity in the proximal surface of the distal abutment tooth. No metal showed in this finished case. The use of a countersunk metal rest in the distal inlay enabled it to be covered from view with light cured direct composite resin applied at the cementation stage. The patient liked the minimal intervention approach in filling his gap. The only reduction of tooth substance required in this case was subtle prefacing of the abutment sides in order to create flat parallel surfaces. By replacing the existing amalgam restoration with a custom formed indirect inlay, tooth substance was preserved, correct space made for the occlusal rest, and an aesthetic improvement achieved.

In the lower jaw, metal display can be obtrusive and the design of the bridge may likewise be modified to advantage not only to conceal the metal but also to restore the abutments in a more aesthetic way. Adhesive bridgework is suitable for lower as well as upper situations.

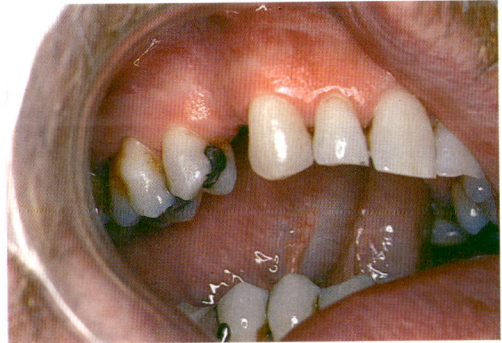

Fig 9-1 Caption: before treatment — note the amalgam filling in the adjacent pre-molar.

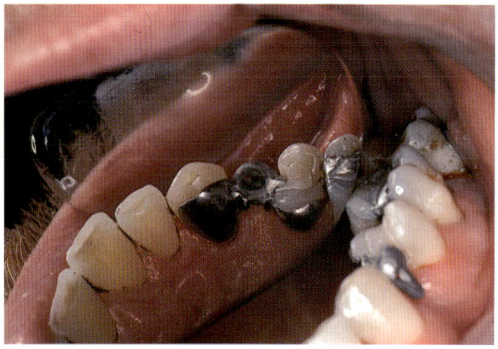

Fig 9-2 Metal try in with inlay; note the countersunk occlusal rest.

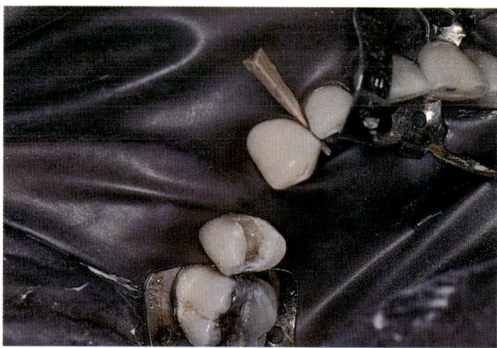

Fig 9-3 Teeth isolated and etched prior to cementation of bridge.

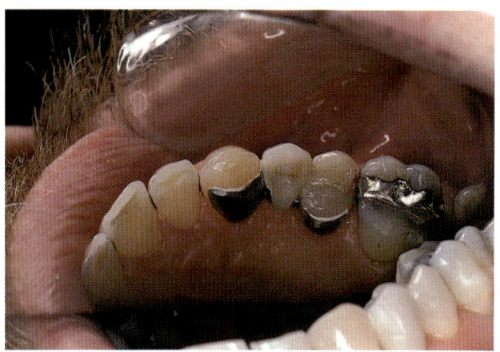

Fig 9-4 Finished bridge.

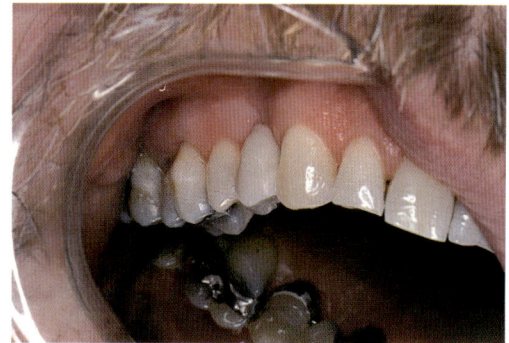

Fig 9-5 No metal is shown.

A middle-aged man shown in Figs 9-6 to 9-12, required the replacement of lower missing teeth. The decision was made to restore this space with the minimum of tooth preparation although this gap could also have been restored with traditional fixed or removable bridgework.

A Maryland design adhesive bridge was chosen, and the molar restored with an indirect resin inlay. One advantage of this method is the ability to use compatible materials in the restoration, and to enable an aesthetic improvement to be made at the same time. The inlay was made with a deep mesial rest that accommodated a counter-sunk metal rest. This rest was then covered with light-cured resin of the same shade. Where it was not possible to countersink the rest, as on the premolar, the metal rest was etched and primed and covered with a thin opaque layer of light cured resin.

At the final clinical appointment the teeth were isolated with rubber dam and the temporary (light cured) inlay removed.

The simple replacement of existing amalgam restorations in the abutment

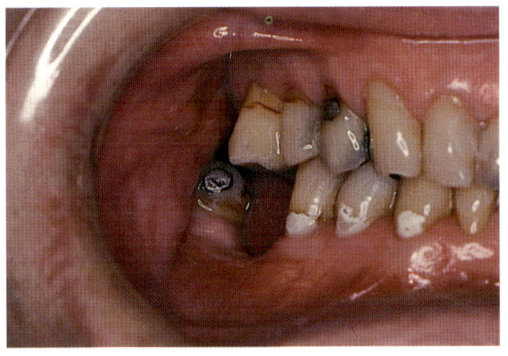

Fig 9-6 Two lower teeth were missing. Reduction of over-erupted upper molar was done following initial occlusal assessment.

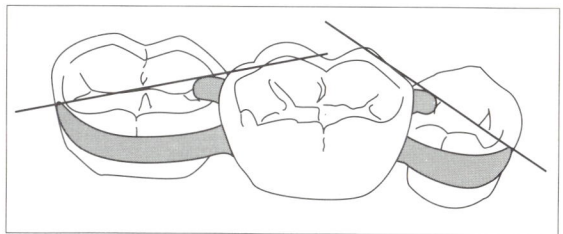

Fig 9-7 The metal framework should extend 180° around the tooth.

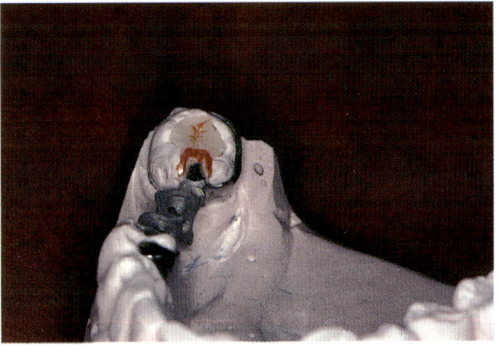

Fig 9-8 Countersunk rest seat outlined in red ink.

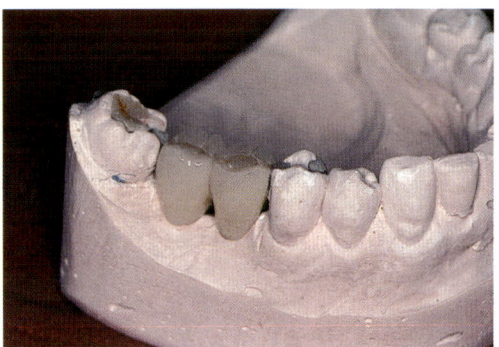

Fig 9-9 Note etched rests.

teeth can greatly improve the final appearance. Here the small buccal filling was replaced with a direct resin using a shade compatible with the indirect inlay and pontics.

Self-curing or dual-curing resin cement is the correct material for use in adhesive bridgework. The abutment teeth are etched and the primed metal undersurface of the bridge will offer good retention for the cured cement. Metal surfaces are chemically and electrolytically etched in the laboratory and must not be contaminated with saliva before cementation.

Following cementation, the surplus cement is trimmed away using a new 12 bladed tungsten carbide bur. The correct finishing of adhesive bridgework should entail fine trimming of the cement and metalwork so that a fine margin of metal with a cement 'halo' is visible. The patient was able to chew again on his right side for the first time in years.

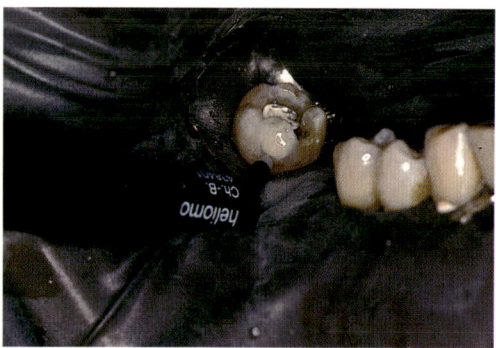

Fig 9-10 The old amalgam is replaced with direct resin.

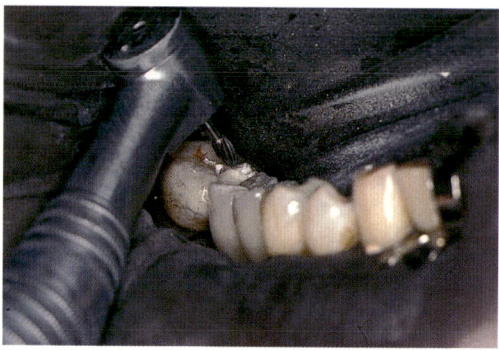

Fig 9-11 Finishing of cement and metalwork.

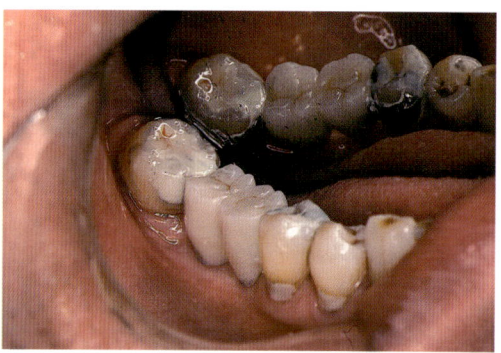

Fig 9-12 The completed bridge.

The versatility of indirect resin material is demonstrated in the case of a middle-aged woman who presented with a missing lower incisor (Fig 9-13). The fractured acid-etched bridge that had carried a pontic was a testament to the inadequacy of this form of treatment. Severe erosion of the remaining incisors posed a restorative problem and the patient was adamant in her wishes to preserve all her remaining teeth.

Following initial prophylaxis and emergency acid-etch work, the case was assessed. Radiographs showed that enough bone support was available to keep the incisors although the extreme erosion was an obstacle to vital full crown preparations. All the teeth were both vital and nonsymptomatic and, in addition, periodontal condition was good.

The most conservative and nondestructive method was chosen. A Maryland bridge was made to restore the missing tooth. Indirect resin veneers were made to restore the incisors and these were matched to the indirect resin pontic on the bridge (Figs 9-13 to 9-17).

In this way the missing tooth was restored and some measure of support given to the remaining teeth, both buccally and lingually. The patient was delighted with her new teeth, and could bite more firmly than before.

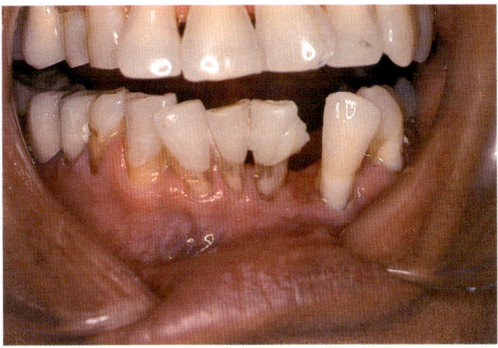

Fig 9-13 Patient presented with missing tooth.

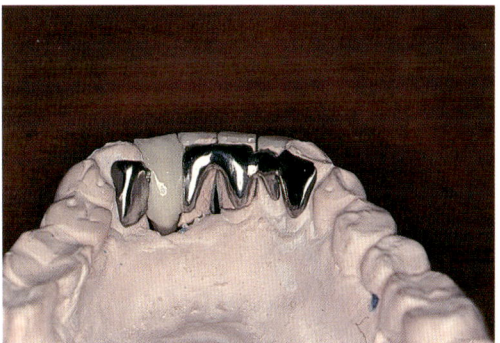

Fig 9-14 Adhesive bridge with single pontic of indirect resin.

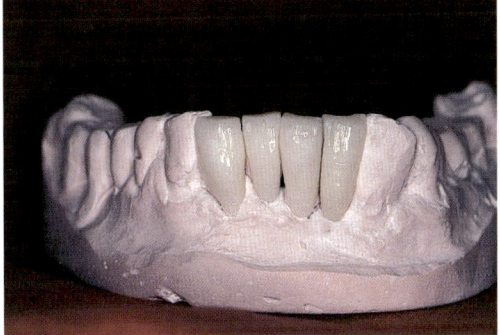

Fig 9-15 Matched veneers and pontic of indirect resin.

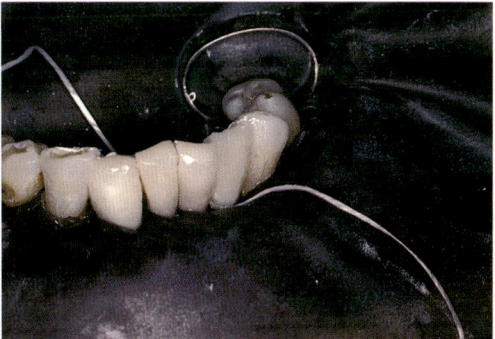

Fig 9-16 Veneers and bridgework attached.

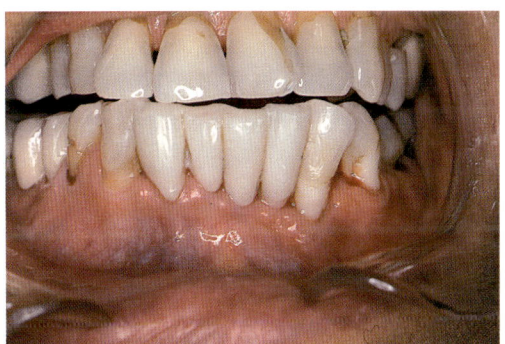

Fig 9-17 Completed case.

Adhesive bridgework is now a well documented and researched method of restoring missing teeth. It is important to understand the principles governing preparation otherwise failure can occur.[5]

References

1   Howe, D.F. and Denehy, G.E. (1977) Anterior fixed partial dentures utilizing the acid-etch technique and a cast metal framework. J. Prosthet. Dent. 37 : 28-31.

2   Livaditis, G.J. (1980) Cast metal resin bonded retainers for posterior teeth. JADA, 101 : 926-929.

3   Livaditis, G.J. (1982) Resin-bonded restoration: preparation of the abutment teeth. Accepted for publication by Int. J. Periodontics & Restorative Dent. May.

4   Gratton, D.R., McConnell, R.J., Jordan, R.E., Suzuki, M. and Boksman, L. (1986) Observations on the clinical performance of resin bonded bridges. J. Dent. Res., 65 : 533 (Abstract 22).

5   Pegoraro, L.F. and Barrack, G. (1987) A comparison of bond strengths of adhesive cast restorations using different designs, bonding agents, and luting resins. J. Prosthet. Dent. 57 : 133-138.

Chapter 10

Implant Dentistry

Implant supported prosthetics are now accepted as a reliable and predictable method of restoring missing teeth. Studies are constantly being conducted to assess the effectiveness of implant supported prostheses and as more data becomes available it is becoming apparent that this treatment modality is at least as successful, if not more successful than traditional alternatives. One recent study reported that 48 out of 49 edentulous arches restored using implants remained in good function after periods of 5-10 years.

With regard to the aesthetic aspects of implant restorations, it should, however, be borne in mind that a combination of factors often conspire to dictate a less than ideal result. It will be shown, using clinical examples, how indirect resins can improve aesthetics. The changes that occur following tooth extraction are well known and alveolar remodelling together with associated resorption leads to loss of hard and soft tissues, which both need to be replaced by some type of prosthesis, either fixed or removable.[1][2]

This situation is frequently worsened by previous chronic periodontal disease around the teeth that were eventually removed. The amount of bone loss may therefore often be severe and even if there is sufficient bone remaining to allow implants to be placed, there will necessarily be an amount of hard and soft tissue to be replaced with the prosthesis. This type of implant supported prosthesis must combine teeth with artificial soft tissue (gum-work) and so needs to be detachable.

Examples of how it is possible, nevertheless, to secure satisfactory results without aesthetic compromise will be shown in the following three cases.

Example 1

Single tooth replacement
A 30 year old patient needed extraction of a hopelessly carious upper canine tooth. Note the interdental spacing that prevented a fixed bridge from being prescribed (Fig 10-1). A root-form ceramic implant (CBS) was placed shortly after removal of the tooth and allowed to osseo-integrate.

The rationale for selecting this type of implant and placing it at an early stage was to retain the maximum bone height and gingival attachment. The placement of an implant can arrest bone resorption and is documented as a method of preserving bone height. Following a period of healing without any occlusal forces, a treatment crown of indirect resin was made in the fifth month. A treatment crown is a crown made to fulfil a particular purpose during the patient's treatment but not necessarily designed for long term use. An example of a treatment crown, or bridge, would be during the making of an anterior bridge where appearance, speech and occlusion would need to be checked before making the final restoration.

Treatment crowns are frequently used in implant prosthetics when an interim period of controlled loading is required. In an area where bone quality is less than ideal, this phase of 'Progressive Bone Loading' (Misch) can make the difference between success and failure.

In this region of the mouth, where occlusal stresses can be great, the danger of implant failure is magnified and special precautions need to be taken to prevent the overloading of the implant. Again, indirect resin is a suitable material to select, as it permits articulation to be finalised in the mouth and wears at a rate comparable to the other teeth.

Canine guidance is absolutely contra-indicated in this case, and the crown was articulated into group function with the other teeth.

Caution

Successful implant dentistry can certainly be incorporated into a general restorative practice, but it requires a careful interpretation of the basic principles that govern osseo-integration. However, no materials can compensate for poor technique.

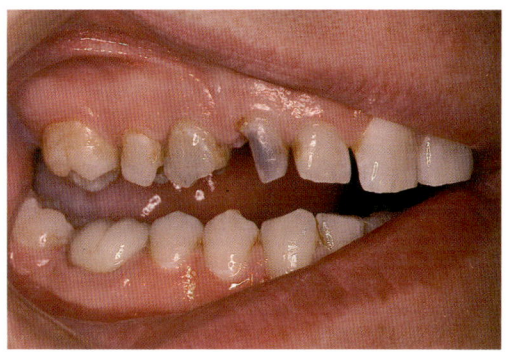

Fig 10-1 Upper canine (cuspid) required extraction.

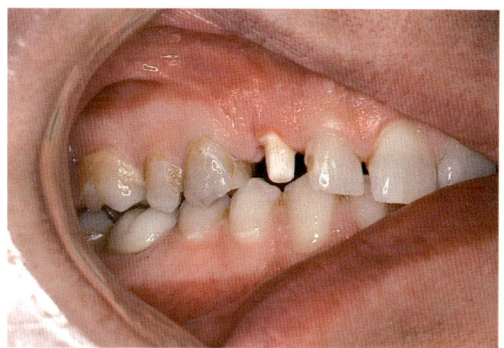

Fig 10-2 Implant shortly after placement.

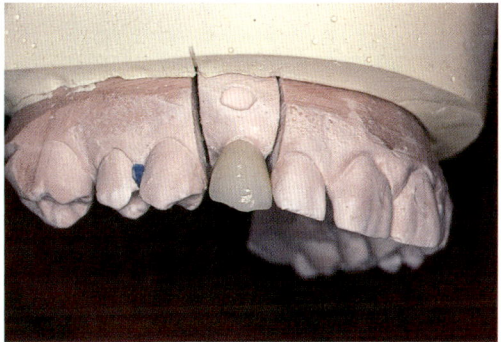

Fig 10-3 Treatment crown of indirect resin.

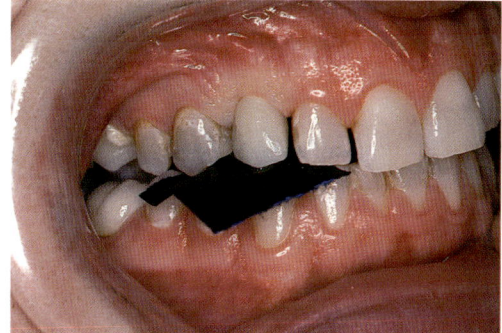

Fig 10-4 Group function obtained.

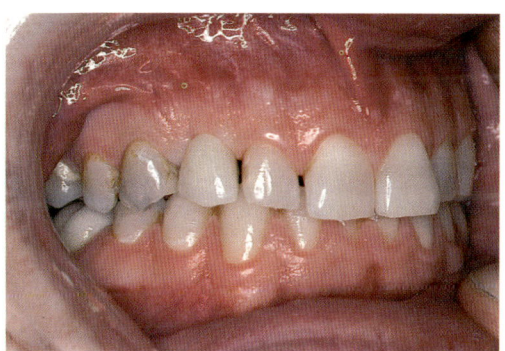

Fig 10-5 Treatment crown functioning in harmony; the natural spacing between teeth has not been disturbed and an aesthetic result obtained.

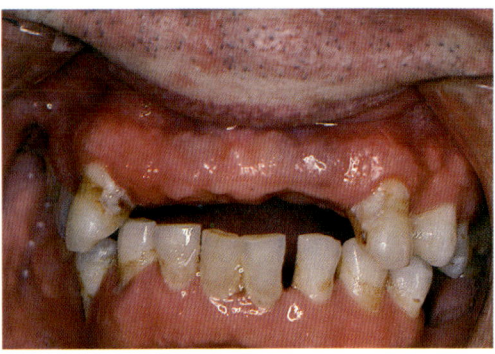

Fig 10-6 The adverse distal inclination, coupled with short clinical crowns of both canines/cuspids. Note poor oral hygiene.

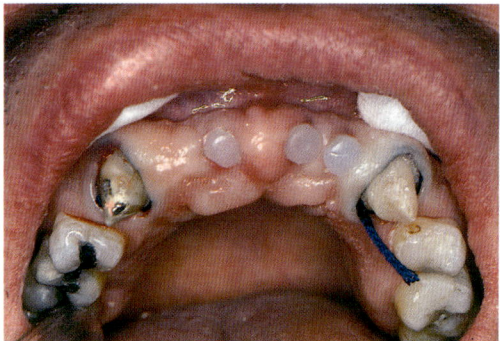

Fig 10-7 Healing caps in position.

Example 2

Multiple tooth replacement
Indirect resin is also suitable for multiple implant restorations both anteriorly and posteriorly. An example of an anterior case is shown in Figs 10-6 to 10-12. This 56 year old man requested fixed replacement of his missing upper incisors. The adverse inclination of the canines (cuspids) and their short clinical crowns prevented fixed bridgework from being selected as the treatment of choice. Following oral hygiene improvements, three implants (screw vent) were placed and allowed to osseo-integrate.

This example illustrates the versatility of indirect resin which may be formed to restore teeth in an aesthetic way when the implant position is less than ideal. Available bone and anatomical considerations frequently determine implant position, and these may not coincide with optimal aesthetics. Interproximal

and other contours can easily be tailored at the chairside and repolished to a high lustre when fused porcelain would need to be returned to the laboratory for re-glazing. Indirect resin anterior teeth should be backed and supported with a metal substructure. Fig 10-9 shows the palatal view on the model.

Nowhere is attention to occlusion more important than with implant work. Implants lack the periodontal membrane and movement potential of natural teeth, and have an ankylosed attachment to bone. Any adverse occlusal forces acting on implants are likely to result in eventual failure.

This case shows that an entire metal palatal surface is desirable in order to establish and maintain a satisfactory anterior guidance. The patient was pleased with his new smile, and a change in his marital status soon followed the completion of treatment.

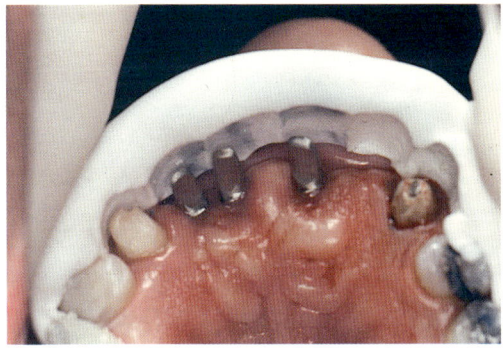

Fig 10-8 The inter-root dimension allowed three implants to be placed. The labial mask was used as a check to ensure that each post lay within the desired position for the new crowns.

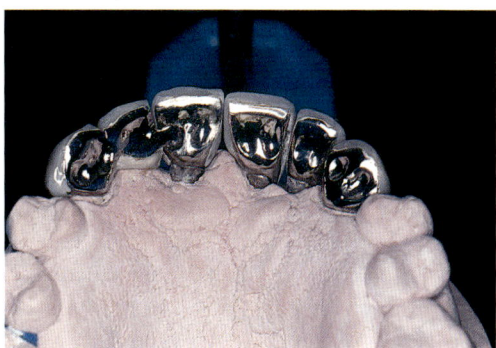

Fig 10-9 A cantilever pontic was made to replace the upper right lateral incisor; note the rest on the implant retained central incisor.

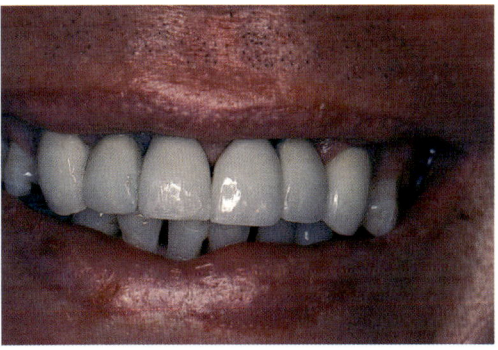

Fig 10-10 The patient's smile line does not reveal the implant/crown margins. An assessment of the position of smile line is an important part of all pre-aesthetic dentistry.

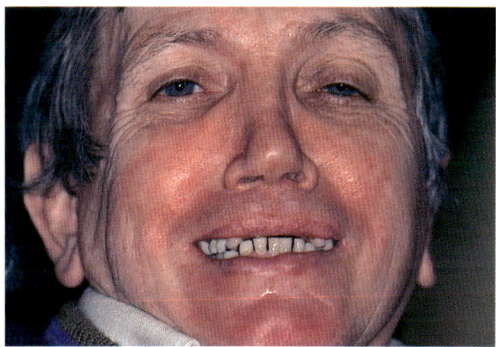

Fig 10-11 Before treatment.

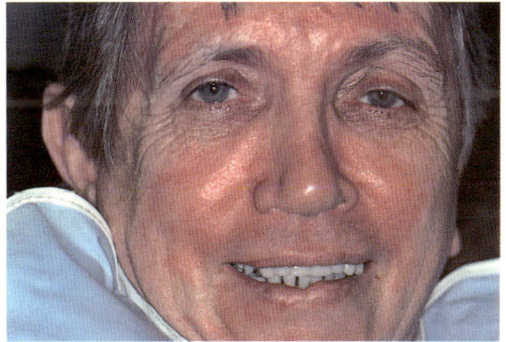

Fig 10-12 After completed restoration.

Example 3

Indirect resins possess two further physical qualities that are assets in implant restorations. The resin material is resilient and may allow some shock-absorption which could compensate for the lack of any periodontal apparatus around the implants. Indirect resin also wears at approximately 7 microns per year and this can be an advantage when considering the dangers of differential wear between natural and artificial teeth, which can result in greater occlusal forces and possible implant failure. Glazed porcelain shows no appreciable wear and could result in excessive occlusal forces after some time.[3]

Posterior teeth replacement
The use of indirect resin teeth in a posterior situation is illustrated in Figs 10-13 to 10-17. This patient was so comfortable with his upper implant supported teeth that he wanted to dispense with his lower denture and have fixed lower teeth as well.

Two basket design implants (core vent) were placed and allowed to osseo-integrate. Joined metal castings were made to fit precisely onto the posts. The metal work substructure allowed for entire occlusal coverage with resin.

As an alternative, the occlusion could have been formed in gold. Note the retention beads which ensure a secure bonding of the resin together with a chemical bonding agent (Spectra-link). It is always advisable to try in the metalwork and at this stage an accurate inter-occlusal record can be made with the natural teeth in contact.

The final prosthetics is then tried in and careful articulation performed so that no adverse occlusal forces could act on these teeth. Ideally there should be no contact in any lateral occlusion.

Indirect resin is also useful in detachable prostheses which can be formed to resemble teeth and also supporting tissues. The technical and laboratory demands of implant dentistry are even more stringent than for conventional crown and bridgework, as implants do not possess even the slight leeway that periodontal ligaments around natural teeth provide.

The indirect resin technique is a welcome partner in aiding precise implant prosthetics.

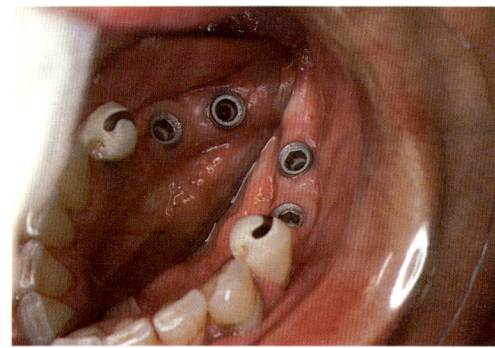

Fig 10-13 Two basket design implants after osseo-integration (Core-vent).

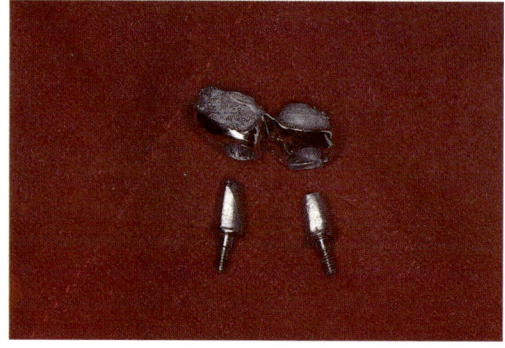

Fig 10-14 Joined metal castings were made to fit precisely on to the posts.

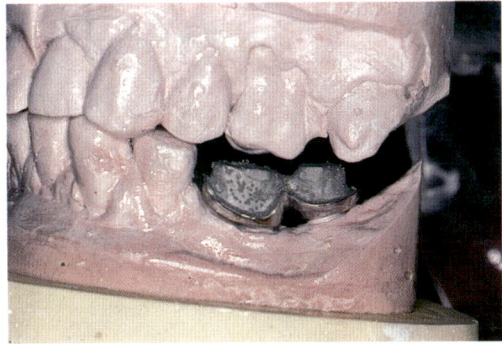

Fig 10-15 Note retention beads on casting surface.

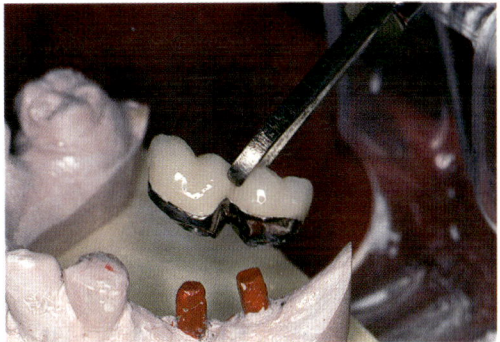

Fig 10-16 Crowns ready for fitting.

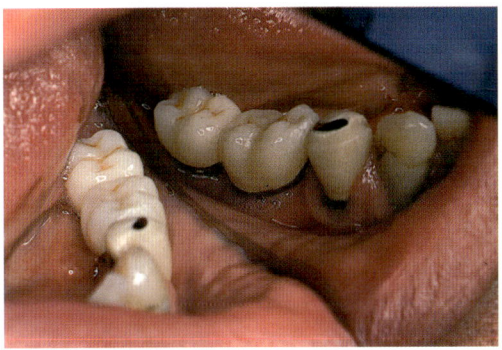

Fig 10-17 The finished restorations.

References

1 Stein, R.S. (1965) Pontic-residual bridge relationship, a research report. J. Prosthet. Dent. 16:251.
2 Watson, R.M., Forman, G.H. and Welfore, R.D. (1988) Essentials of case planning for osseointegrated implants. Brit. Dent. J., pp.313, 21 May.
3 Davis, D.M., Rimrott, Robert and Zarbga. (1988) The effects of adding composite, acrylic or porcelain on implant structures. Int. J. of Oral and Maxillo-Facial Implants, pp.275-280.

Suggested further reading

Parel and Sullivan. (1989) Esthetics and osseointegration. Taylor Co.

Conclusion

The examples illustrated and described in this book amply demonstrate that indirect resin should have its place as a unique restorative material and thus end any confusion as to its role in modern dentistry. Some practitioners have already found many useful applications, whilst others may not have realised its full potential.

The advent of a new restorative material sometimes heralds the demise of an old one and in this context mention may be made of acrylic resin, which nowadays has little to commend it in restorative dentistry. More frequently, a new material carves a niche for itself and offers a different way of achieving treatment objectives. Indirect resin can, therefore, be more suitable than light-cured resin in some teeth but not others: each case now has to be assessed with a background knowledge of the properties of both types of material. Another example is where either a porcelain inlay, onlay or veneer is an alternative treatment option. Again, the choice should be made from a position of knowledge, not dogma.

Indirect resin is not a universal wonder material, and like any material can fail if used outside of its physical abilities. The author believes that the cases presented in this book show how this material does offer real advantages in many situations and contends that the progressive dentist should consider indirect resin seriously.

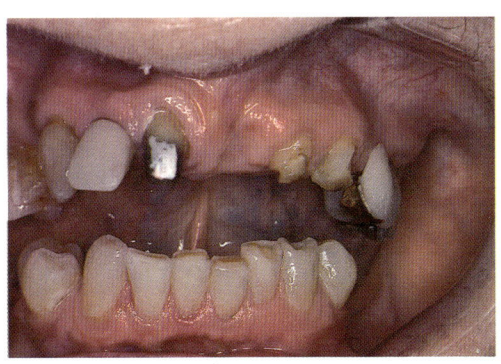

Fig 11-1 An elderly patient presented with considerable problems.

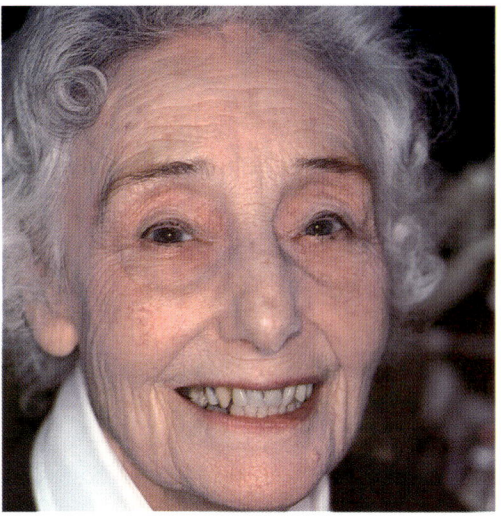

Fig 11-2 The patient after successful treatment with a blend of crowns and removable prostheses both utilizing indirect resin.

Some Questions Answered

The author has found that those who have not yet used an indirect resin system often raise questions which they would like answered.

This short section seeks to provide answers to those questions which are most frequently asked.

I am able to produce good direct restorations in most situations, so why do I need to use Indirect resins?

Indirect resins do not supercede direct resins. There are clinical indications and merits for both types, which are distinct. Direct resin restorations are more suited to smaller cavity designs, in anterior and premolar teeth. These teeth usually have less occlusal loading than molars, and direct composite resins have proved satisfactory over reasonable periods of time.

Direct resin is also indicated in situations where cavity design or pre-existing undercuts would require the inordinate removal of tooth structure so that proper draw could be established for an inlay. Indirect techniques are more suited to larger cavities in any tooth that needs aesthetic and structural repair. Cuspal coverage is easy to provide and studies have demonstrated that indirect resins wear less than any direct restoration that was tested.

Although I have not yet started using aesthetic inlays or onlays, my understanding from the literature is that porcelain would be a superior material for achieving good appearance with longevity.

The porcelains available until recently were based on traditional crown and bridge porcelain and certainly cannot be bettered when correctly executed in the right situations.

However the technique is critical and not as easy to master as the indirect resin method. A recent comparison study by the American Academy of Esthetic Dentistry found that more porcelain than resin inlays had failed.

Newer porcelain materials are now being introduced, and they are expected to overcome many of the difficulties encountered with the traditional porcelains.

I often notice a white line around the margins of my direct composite fillings after finishing. Can I expect the same unaesthetic border around indirect inlays?

White lines are avoidable in both direct

and indirect resins. White lines are in fact the visible result of damage to the marginal enamel prisms. This can occur during cavity preparation but is usually caused by careless finishing of the resin margins with blunt burs and a heavy hand.

Careful finishing of all resin-etched fillings should prevent white lines.

I often encounter post-operative sensitivity complaints from patients who have had resin restorations placed in vital teeth. The teeth are sensitive to temperature changes and sometimes to pressure as well. Is this likely to happen when I embark on indirect resins as well?

There are two kinds of post-operative sensitivity: temperature and pressure, and it is suspected that these problems have different causes.

Temperature sensitivity may be due to pulpal irritation from etching acid, whereas pressure sensitivity can result from stresses within the tooth that occur following polymerisation shrinkage.

Both these unwelcome side-effects can be prevented by following the correct placement protocol for indirect resins.

Pulpal irritation will be prevented if an adequate lining and dentine adhesive (or protection) is applied.

Polymerisation shrinkage is minimised in the Indirect method, as this takes place in the technician's laboratory. The onlay polymerisation shrinkage that takes place in the tooth is that of the resin cement.

I find it easier to design cavity preparations when I have some numerical data on the ideal proportions.

Cavity dimensions are well documented for gold inlays, but these designs are not appropriate for resin materials which possess different physical properties.

It is important to avoid thin sections at any portion of the final inlay or onlay. Veneers are excepted from this rule.

A guide might be to allow the maximum thickness possible and not to have final sections less than 1.5mm. Cusps should be covered with 1.5 to 2mm of resin, and occlusal sections should be at least 2mm deep.

I find that the delicate margins of my inlays split off as I try in the inlays; does this not mean that the system is flawed?

No. You, or your technician, have failed to understand that resin inlay preparations should not follow traditional gold inlay designs. Bevelled margins are not desirable, and a passive fit of inlays is correct. The margin should be a butt fit, and there should be no overhang of resin onto the tooth.

I have trouble seating inlays, they are sometimes tight and require easing; can this be avoided?

The most common cause of tight fit is polymerisation shrinkage during the laboratory curing process. All resin materials contract during curing, and this has been measured in tests to be between 1 and 2%.

The technician should ease inlays by selective grinding to ensure a passive fit on the model. Failure to do this will result in an inlay which will not fit on the model or in the mouth. Shrinkage is not linear, and depends upon the geometry of each individual cavity, but is often apparent on the axial sides of proximal boxes.

The technician can resort to the use of a compatible die spacer to overcome this.

I find recurrent caries at the base of some direct resin class two fillings. Is this undesirable complication liable to occur with indirect resins as well?

Two factors can permit recurrent caries at the base of direct resin fillings.

Polymerisation contraction has been studied and documented to occur near the gingival margins of boxes, leading to open margins. Secondly, light curing of direct resins is sometimes incomplete, and the areas furthest from the occlusal parts are most affected. These problems are overcome in the Indirect system.

Polymerisation occurs in the laboratory, and the final restorations are then cemented with a resin cement that has a film thickness of less than 100 microns.

The contraction of a thin film of resin cement is very much less than when an entire resin filling is cured.

The cement is dual curing, but it will not completely cure in the absence of light. The danger of uncured margins can be avoided if adequate initial light curing is made. (See Chapter 2.)

My patients have experienced fractures of indirect resin after some time. Can this be avoided?

Indirect resin is strong enough to resist fracture in normal occlusions, provided that there is adequate bulk of material. Thin veneers should be avoided at all times, and the maximum thickness possible made.

As in all restorative dentistry, a pre-operative assessment of the occlusion should be carried out. Resin materials are not indicated in areas of very high stress. Bruxism is one example.

Appendix: Technical Aspects

Laboratory Procedures

Most manufacturers of indirect resin systems provide special training courses both for dentists and for the staff of dental laboratories producing restorations using these materials.

This appendix is not, in any way, intended as a substitute for such courses but readers may find it helpful to have an outline understanding of laboratory procedures used in producing restorations with Isosit indirect resin materials.

Intra-Coronal Restorations

The elastomeric impression of the prepared tooth, or teeth, is cast twice in hard plaster with one cast made into a split model. Seven basic shades of inlay/onlay are available, corresponding with the shades on the basic shade guide. Laboratories that have completed the training courses offered by the manufacturers will be conversant with the handling of the material and with all the procedures required to produce indirect resin restorations that are ready to fit at the second clinical appointment.

Extra-Coronal Restorations

The extra-coronal crown, bridge and veneer material Chromasit (formerly SR Isosit N) is available in dentine, cervical and incisal formulations. It is designed to be used as a facing over cast metal substructures, which may be precious or non-precious. By the use of both physical and chemical bonding, secure retention to the metal base is provided. It is also designed for forming laminate veneers.

Colour

The basic colour is derived from the dentine shades: there are 20 shades of dentine that correspond to the appropriate shade guide (Chromoscop).

Technicians who have completed training will be fully conversant with all the laboratory procedures necessary to create resin bonded to metal restorations ready for fitting. A special opaqing system (Spectrasit) is a necessary part of the process. This material ensures complete masking of metal sub-structures, and should be utilised in all cases. The Spectrasit system of physio-chemical bonding is also used to enhance attachment of resin to metal.

Veneers

Indirect resin laminate veneers are made using extra-coronal resin (Chromasit) in a layering method that permits internal colouration to be introduced.

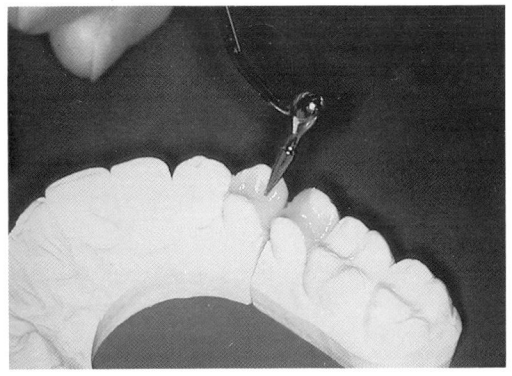

T1 Inlays being formed on model.

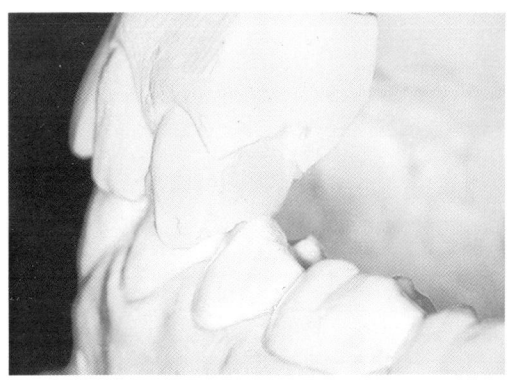

T2 The occlusion is checked.

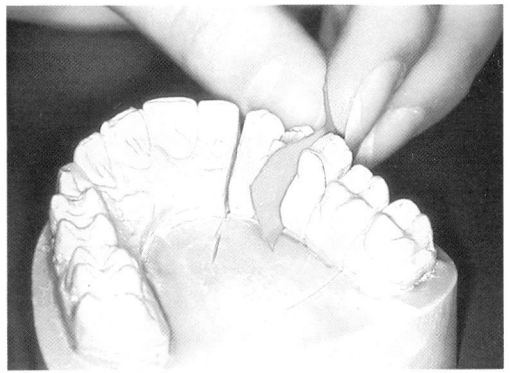

T3 The contacts are checked.

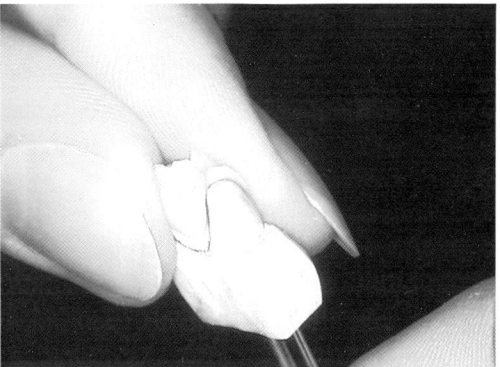

T4 The inlays are examined for marginal fit.

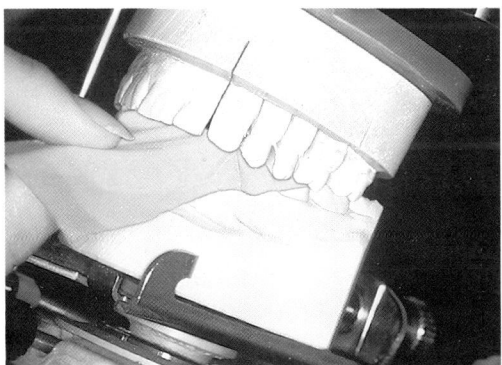

T5 The occlusion is checked.

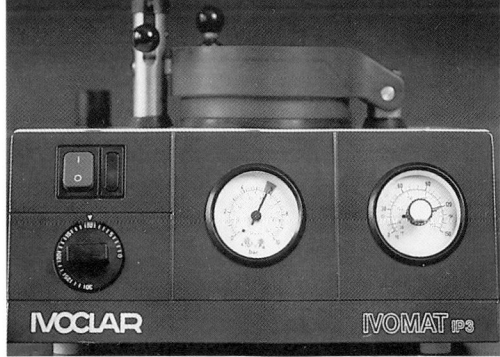

T6 Specially designed temperature and pressure vessel for curing.

Systematic Shade Selection

The same shade guide (Chromascop) is required to convey appropriate information to the technician whenever the extra-coronal material is chosen. This shade system is also compatible with resin and porcelain denture teeth of the same make.

For accurate rendering of shades the use of a contemporary mapping device is recommended (Colour Palette). This is very helpful to the technician, who is then able to construct crowns and veneers to the precise requirements of each case.

Dentine Adhesive

Syntac is a two phase adhesive system to ensure adhesion between composite resin and enamel dentine. The low film thickness does not inhibit the fit of the inlay/onlay during cementation.

> *Composition*
> Primer: Aliphathic dimethacrylate in acidic acetone water.
> Adhesive: a dimethacrylate and a dialdehyde solution in water.
>
> *Film thickness:* 10 microns.
>
> High early bonding capability.

Resin Activator

Special Bond II is a light curing resin bonding agent designed to enhance bonding of indirect resins and veneers to resin cement. This is necessary wherever laminate veneers are being fitted and is optional when fitting inlays and onlays.

Lining Material

Basic-1 is a two paste presentation, light cured lining material which is radio opaque.

> *Composition:* Calcium hydroxide base paste with organic additives. Activator paste containing barium sulphate and activator ingredients.
>
> Inhibited surface layer of cured material will establish a bond to resin restoratives.

Resin Cement

Dual Cement is a microfilled resin cement in a two-paste presentation. It is light and chemical cured and is radio opaque.

> *Composition*
> Base paste: 30% dimethacrylates; 40% silicon dioxide fillers, microfilled; 30% barium trifluoride.
> Catalyst paste: 31% dimethacrylates; 41% silicon dioxide fillers, microfilled; 28% barium trifluoride.

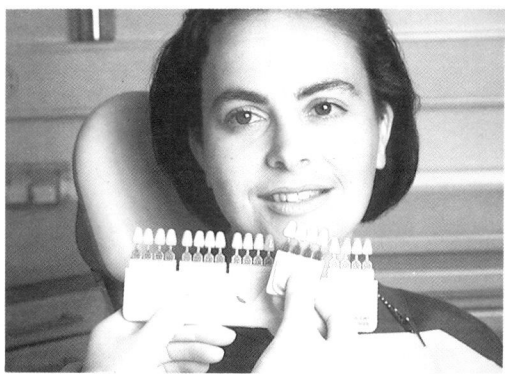

T7 The Chromoscop shade guide for extra-coronal colour matching.

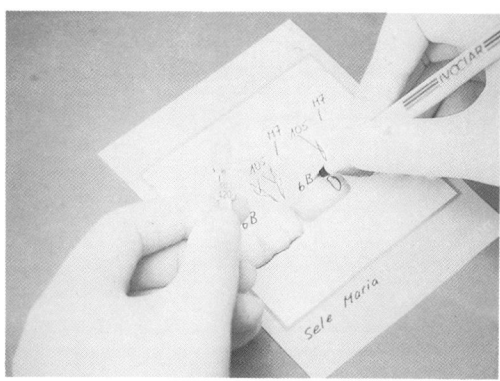

T8 Use of colour palette for accurate colour registration.

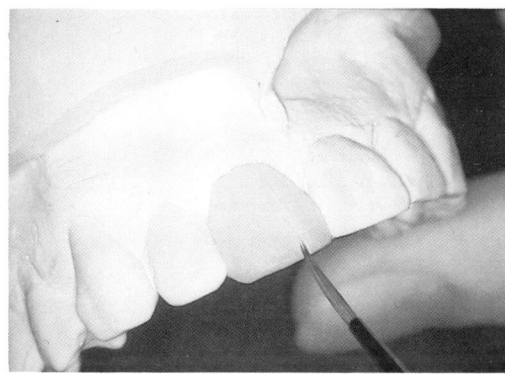

T9 Chromasit being formed into a laminate veneer.

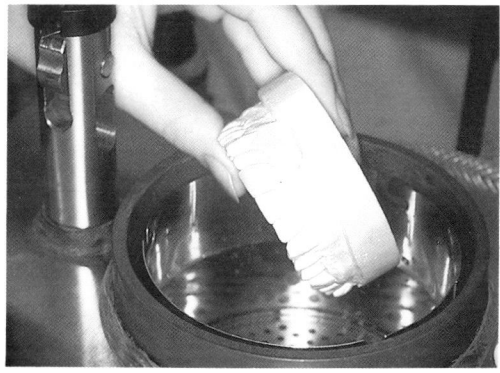

T10 Chromasit veneer is heat/pressure cured in the specially designed vessel.

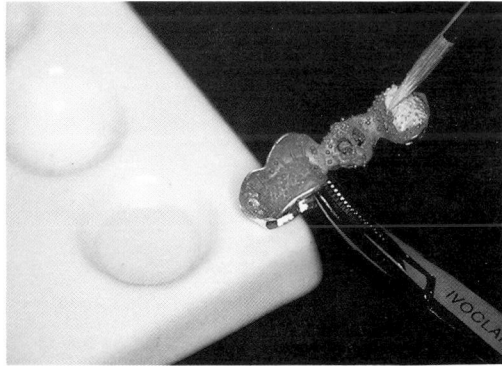

T11 Use of Spectra-link and opaquing resin on metal casting.

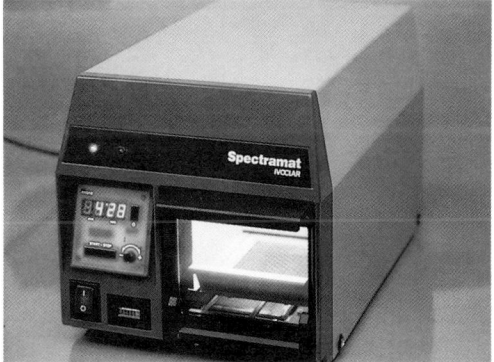

T12 Spectramat equipment used for enhanced bonding.